Praise for *Child's Mind*

"Christopher Willard's delightful book *Child's Mind* makes the wonder and transformative power of mindfulness meditation accessible to everyone. His elegantly simple practices are a joy to read and will impact kids and families for generations to come."

—Susan Kaiser Greenland, author of *The Mindful Child*

"Teaching mindfulness to children sounds great in theory, but really, how do we do it? This wonderful book, chock full of mindfulness practices adapted to children of all ages, is the answer! Christopher Willard offers us skillful advice, illuminating words, and a treasure chest of practices for schools, clinicians, and our own family's kitchen table."

—Diana Winston, Director of Mindfulness Education at the Mindful Awareness Research Center of UCLA and author of *Wide Awake: A Buddhist Guide for Teens*

"This book is an excellent resource for parents, teachers, and health-care providers who want to share the benefits of mindfulness with children. The varied practices are presented with clarity and joy, making them both accessible and engaging."

—Amy Saltzman, M.D., Association for Mindfulness in Education and creator of the *Still Quiet Place* CD series

"As a parent and teacher, I am deeply grateful for Christopher Willard's book. It is an important contribution toward making the practice of meditation an integral part of the school curriculum and, more generally, toward raising healthier, happier children."

—Tal Ben-Shahar, Harvard University, author of *Happier*

"*Child's Mind* is an invitation to raise children who grow up relating to themselves, others, and the world around them with care and compassion. Parents and teachers looking for practical advice for teaching mindfulness to children will find it here."

—Paul R. Fulton, Institute for Meditation and Psychotherapy

"If you're considering how to bring mindfulness into the lives of children, this book is the place to begin. The author offers skillful, detailed exercises designed to entice and reveal. There's something for every child, including those with special challenges. I recommend this book for anyone who wants to be eased into the original wonder and delight of mindfulness practice, or who wants their kids to grow up savoring each precious moment of their lives."

—Christopher K. Germer, Ph.D., Clinical Instructor in Psychology at Harvard Medical School and author of *The Mindful Path to Self-Compassion*

"*Child's Mind* is a wise, creative, and practical collection of exercises for teaching mindfulness to children. Willard's compassion and his skillful translation of meditation practices shine through every page. Every teacher, parent, and therapist will benefit from this book, as will the children in their lives."

—Janet L. Surrey, Ph.D., Institute for Meditation and Psychotherapy, Wellesley College

"This wonderful book suggests simple and fun exercises that lead to profound growth towards joy, calmness, strength, and emotional intelligence. The list of 'A hundred things for kids to do mindfully' is worth the price of this important work. I recommend *Child's Mind* to therapists, educators, parents, and anyone else who wants to help children develop into kind, happy, and resilient human beings."

—Mary Pipher, author *Seeking Peace* and *Reviving Ophelia*

Child's Mind

Mindfulness Practices to Help Our Children Be More Focused, Calm, and Relaxed

Christopher Willard

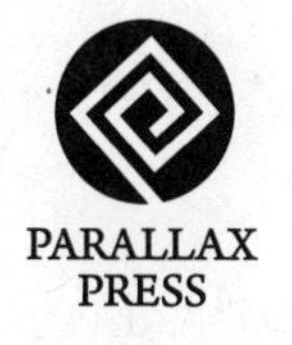

PARALLAX PRESS

Berkeley, California

For parents and children.

For those who heal, and those who are healing.

For those who teach, and those who learn.

And for Chuck.

—Christopher Willard

Parallax Press
P.O. Box 7355
Berkeley, California 94707

Parallax Press is the publishing division of Unified Buddhist Church, Inc.

Printed in the United States of America

Cover design by Robin Terra
Text design by Gopa&Ted2, Inc.
Author photo by Richard Friday

Library of Congress Cataloging-in-Publication Data

Willard, Christopher, Psy. D.
Child's mind : mindfulness practices to help our children be more focused, calm, and relaxed / Christopher Willard.
p. cm.
ISBN 978-1-935209-62-1
1. Meditation for children. 2. Mind and body in children. I. Title.
BF723.M37W55 2010
158.1'2083—dc22

2010021199

3 4 5 / 15 14 13

Contents

Practices

In the beginner's mind, there are many possibilities,
in the expert's mind, there are few.
—Suzuki Roshi

An Invitation

So many of us spend our time rushing around and doing, taking little or no time for just being. This kind of existence has created not just busy adults, but overbooked, overloaded, and anxious children. Children absorb the stresses of the adults in their lives and the stresses of their environment. Stressed out and unbalanced parents and caregivers can unintentionally create stressed out kids. Many children are so busy doing sports, homework, activities, and classes, they have no time to just quietly be with themselves and come to know themselves and the world around them. For many lower-income children, these stresses are compounded by issues of violence, hunger, and poverty. Young people of all backgrounds are spending more and more time with passive entertainment such as portable game systems, cell phones, and televisions rather than actively engaging the world.

Mindfulness practice offers something radically different: an effective path for people of all ages and backgrounds to develop healthy responses to a chaotic world around them and often inside of them. Mindfulness is simple; it doesn't require buying any equipment, carrying any special supplies, or learning anything complicated. It can be taught by a parent, relative, teacher, therapist, or other caregiver, or even by a young person's peer.

How can we convince a child to sit still and meditate, not to mention schedule that time in our own busy lives? This book is not about teaching children to sit in the lotus position for long periods of time. Instead, I suggest short, simple exercises that can plant the seeds of meditative awareness in all aspects of our children's lives. Thich Nhat Hanh, the Vietnamese monk who helped popularize mindfulness practice in the West, advocates transforming everyday life into a meditation, and meditation into a way of life. We can do this by bringing mindful awareness to our breathing, walking, driving, eating, working, and all our simple daily tasks. Children already have a head start on this. They have a natural tendency to notice the details that we adults overlook, ask the questions we've stopped asking, and be open to new experiences without prejudgment.

The exercises in this book are designed for children's diverse attention spans and diverse sensory learning styles. Because the purest water flows closest to the spring, I offer some original meditation techniques that have been used for hundreds of years. These include adaptations of more grown-up practices, some of which have been made into games, art projects, and fun activities.

To get children started with mindfulness, you don't need to be an expert. In fact, mindfulness is something you and the children in your life can learn and practice together. This book aims to help you create or strengthen your own mindfulness practice so that you can effectively share it with the children in your life. Introducing a child to mindfulness practice is a lifelong gift. You are planting the seeds for a practice that can help sustain and nourish mind, body, and spirit for a lifetime.

Planting Seeds

1

Introduction to Mindfulness Meditation

MEDITATION IS increasingly part of Western culture. Zen chic sells computers, cell phones, and cars; the Buddha's image is on everything from T-shirts to key chains; yoga studios sprout like wildflowers; and meditation books occasionally top best-seller lists. Some doctors recommend meditation for everything from heart conditions to insomnia, and many therapists now teach clients breathing exercises to encourage calm and relaxation. Meditation and all things Eastern may be trendy, but the practices and benefits are universal, transcending time, culture, religion, and marketing trends. How many other practices in our culture do religious and scientific minds agree upon?

In my experience teaching mindfulness, anyone—from prisoners and college students to doctors and developmentally delayed children—can respond to mindfulness practices, at least on some level. I've worked with people who refuse outright to even try sitting still and breathing, and yet have left a class or workshop admitting that they feel a little less frustrated. I think this is in part because mindfulness practice doesn't try to "do" anything to you or force you to believe anything, it just invites you to notice where you are, and what is happening, and how you are responding in any given moment. The actual present moment is often a lot less stressful than the stories our minds invent about the past, present, and future.

What Exactly Is Meditation?

Contemplative techniques like mindfulness and concentration meditation have been practiced for thousands of years. There is Transcendental Meditation, mindfulness meditation, Zen meditation, Christian meditation, Kaballah meditation, and insight meditation, to name just a few. Then there are a host of practices like yoga, tai chi, even hypnosis and others that seem to have something to do with meditation, but it's not necessarily clear what.

For this book, I use a definition that is more scientific than spiritual. Meditation is "a practice that self-regulates the body and mind, thereby affecting mental events by engaging a specific attentional set. These practices are a subset of those used to induce relaxation or states such as hypnosis, progressive relaxation, and trance."[1]

Although this definition is very dry, it captures an important essence of meditation. Another way to put it is this: Meditation is a practice of focusing one's attention that affects both mind and body. I like this description because it reminds us meditation is an active process, correcting the common misconception that meditation is somehow passive. The focus on attention contradicts the misconception that meditation is an attempt to stop or block your thoughts. In fact, when you begin to meditate you will notice lots of thoughts rushing in. The trick is to let these thoughts float past you, without getting "stuck" on any particular one. In this way, meditation is an exercise of training the mind that allows us to see our own thought patterns more clearly.

Sometimes people worry that meditation, with its emphasis on acceptance, will make them more passive or turn them into a pushover or a doormat. This is a fundamental misinterpretation of mindful acceptance. With practice, we learn to see our situation more clearly and then have the wisdom of knowing when and how to act.

I often respond to people's concern about meditation's passivity by describing a scientific study that looked specifically at the physical signs of anxiety in three groups: meditators, non-meditators, and new meditators, all of whom were watching film clips of car accidents—hardly relaxing! Each group became equally stressed—that is, their temperature, blood pressure, heart rate, and other physiological signs of stress increased about the same amount before and during the accidents they watched. But the groups who meditated recovered faster from the stress, returning to baseline long before the non-meditators.[2] These results suggest that meditators bounce back faster and may even be more resilient when they have difficult experiences. Of course meditators experience stress, worry, and fear like everyone else. Rather than passively ignoring these feelings, they seem to be able to actively experience them without letting these feelings linger or interfere with their lives. Most people I've spoken to who have started practicing meditation describe feeling more actively engaged in life, not less.

Forms of Meditation

Traditional and contemporary meditation teachers typically divide meditation into two major types: concentration meditation and mindfulness meditation. In Pali, the language of many of the earliest Buddhist texts, these are known as *samadhi* (concentration) practices and *sati* (mindfulness) practices.

Concentration is single-pointed awareness; the focus of attention is on one thing, either internal or external, for a duration of time.[3] External objects of awareness could include viewing a candle, contemplating beautiful artwork, or simply gazing at a spot on the wall. The focus on internal objects could include visualizing an image, breathing, noting body sensations or following movements, or repeating a mantra. A mantra is a simple word like "one," "peace," or "love" or a sound like "*om*" that is meaningful to the person repeating it. "Om" is a sound often heard in Eastern traditions; in Hinduism it is believed to be the original divine vibration of the universe. As mental or physical distractions arise, they are simply set aside and attention is redirected at the object of concentration. Commonly known concentration meditations can include yoga, tai chi, qigong, as well as Transcendental Meditation and other focused tasks, including many types of prayer that may be more familiar to many Westerners. Buddhist concentration meditation includes practices like *metta* (a loving kindness meditation) as well as some Zen and many Tibetan meditations. Concentration meditation builds attention and clears and calms the mind. It's like traveling to a destination in a straight line.

The practices in this book mostly fall under the large heading called "mindfulness meditation." Mindfulness meditation springs out of the

Zen and Vipassana Buddhist traditions. Unlike concentration meditation, in which we direct our mind where to go, mindfulness practice focuses on observing where the mind goes naturally.[4] If concentration meditation is comparable to a zoom lens upon an object, mindfulness is like a wide-angle lens focused on the whole horizon.[5] Mindfulness brings attention directly to the whole present-moment experience—our perceptions and, perhaps more importantly, the stories our minds make out of them.

Mindfulness meditation involves practicing meta-awareness of thoughts, feelings, and sensations in the present moment. "Meta-awareness" is a term for watching our thoughts without judgment, analysis, or storytelling. We simply note observations about the mind's current activities as thoughts, sensations, and associations that both come and go.[6]

Though the purest mindfulness meditation is simply observing the mind and watching thoughts form and un-form likes clouds in the sky, it is easy for the mind to drift away on a stream of thought. For that reason, it can help to anchor ourselves in a concentration or awareness task to return to, such as following our breath or noticing bodily sensations. As with concentration meditation, there are inevitable distractions or wanderings of the mind with mindfulness meditation that we mentally set aside before refocusing.

In anchored mindfulness meditation, we observe and then simply label a thought, feeling, or sensation before returning our attention to the anchor task. For example, as we focus on our breath for an anchor, we notice the belly growls and suddenly we are swept away in planning dinner. When we notice that, we simply note "stomach growling" and return to the breath, cutting off more of the narrative about planning dinner each time. The practices of observation and coming to know our minds more intimately give us insight into the very nature of our mind and its habits.

Because young people tend to do best with strong anchors and concrete ideas they can see or feel, many of the practices in this book are sensory, honing awareness through the five senses to build a connection to the present moment and to observing the ways we habitually respond. The five senses of hearing, sight, touch, taste, and smell can each be an anchor for our meditation. Some Eastern psychological traditions also include a sixth sense, the mind or thought sense.

Mindfulness Practice

Psychologist Christopher Germer describes mindfulness as "an awareness of present moment experience with acceptance."[7] This is the very awareness and curiosity with which children often view the world. If this definition works for you, use it. If not, here are some common metaphors that may be helpful when thinking about how to describe mindfulness to children. I'm partial to the metaphor of sitting by a stream and watching thoughts carried gently downstream on leaves or boats. The longer we sit by the side of the stream, the more we begin to see what's under the surface and understand the currents as well. But here are a few other ideas:

* Watching a spring or fountain bubble up with thoughts that trickle away
* Thoughts and events carried past on a conveyer belt
* Thoughts marked on signs carried by marchers in a parade
* Thoughts as autumn leaves landing softly on an empty and accepting blanket
* Following the bouncing ball of thought or perception as in old TV sing-alongs or karaoke
* Thoughts as clouds, forming, dissolving, and reforming in the sky, then blowing away
* Sitting on a train looking out the window (rather than climbing out every time you see something interesting)

I also like to think of a chalkboard or whiteboard as the field of consciousness, and meditation as cleaning the board, a classroom chore that a lot of kids tend to enjoy. By the end of the day, the board has been erased over and over, leaving smudges and bits of chalk. Meditation is when we clean our chalkboard, wiping the field of consciousness clear. With mindfulness meditation, we notice each faded word or diagram underneath the day's lessons before wiping it away. Demonstrating this with an actual chalkboard makes a great visual metaphor for children and adults alike.

How Do Meditation and Mindfulness Work?

For years, it was believed that the brain changes little after it stops growing in adolescence. Recently, science has found that the brain is far more flexible. Through meditation and other activities, we can improve what were once thought to be innate and unchangeable qualities like attention, intelligence, and even mental health by essentially rewiring neural connections. As with training the body, we can build strength where we once were weak, though we cannot change our height or shape beyond certain limits. Studies have found, however, that long-term meditators show changes in baseline activity levels in various parts of the brain, and even change the amount and shape of brain gray matter.[8]

Mindfulness trains us to become aware of the nature of mind through noticing our own thought patterns. Mindfulness also changes how we respond to these thoughts or events, and then literally changes the way we think. With practice, the thought patterns we may have lived with our entire lives begin to shift, even on the molecular level.

The body is also affected by meditation. As the mind relaxes, the physical body relaxes, shifting the body to a natural state of healing.[9] When in this state, our mind and body recover more quickly from stress and strain. Body-based meditations can also help us better listen to our body, know when something is wrong, and respond appropriately. Laboratory studies have found that during meditation, our heart rate and blood pressure decline.

Mindfulness activates the areas of the brain associated with healthy regulation of emotions, happiness and a positive outlook, as well as physical and mental resiliency.[10] Because of this, meditation can help with handling strong emotions, seems to create happiness or optimism, and can even strengthen the immune system. Studies have shown that the bodies of meditators recover faster from skin conditions like psoriasis[11] and create more flu antibodies when exposed to vaccines.[12]

Meditation and Children

All of the physical and emotional benefits of mindfulness meditation for adults are applicable to children. Meditation and mindfulness practices can improve and build on children's existing strengths. Meditation is completely natural with no known negative side effects and plenty of benefits for mind, body, brain, and spirit.

Because meditation is an activity that children can improvise and do for themselves, it is fundamentally empowering. Children learn powerful techniques they can use to soothe themselves when upset, focus when they need to, and just be comfortable and awake in the world.

I worked a few years ago with a young woman named Carrie who had struggled for years with Attention Deficit Hyperactivity Disorder (ADHD) and anxiety, trying various medications, therapists, and tutors, all of which helped some, but also sent her the message that there was something wrong with her that only something or someone outside of her could change. Finally, a teacher suggested meditation as a way to help her focus and calm herself down. Carrie had been studying and practicing what she'd learned for a few years before I even met her. She had the confident and self-assured air of a successful student-athlete, a stark contrast to how she described her younger self.

Carrie's parents at first objected to her trying meditation; they thought it was contrary to their religion. However, Carrie's parents came around when they saw that what Carrie was doing was more helpful to her than a lot of other things they had tried and that practicing mindfulness meditation doesn't have to have any particular religious component.

She said, "Okay, so I know everyone thinks it's weird that I do this meditation thing, my friends and definitely my parents at first. I still don't tell everyone, because you never know how people will feel about it. But I've told some of my closer friends recently, and they think it is pretty cool and asked me to teach them." Having kids teach each other these practices also deepens their understanding and sustains their practice.

Carrie put it best as she slouched comfortably in her chair, brown hair still tousled from being under her hockey helmet earlier: "Meditation is mine. It helps me to stay calm and I know it's helped me with focusing on school and on hockey. But it's not a pill that my doctor gives me that changes me, it's *me* and what *I* do that changes me and it's something I can do whenever and wherever I want to. And other people don't have to know that I'm doing it, but if I do share about how it has helped I can really help other people."

2

Meditation Basics

What moments from your own childhood were the most joyful? What do you miss the most? What did you find overwhelming or frightening? What might have helped? What wisdom have you learned as an adult that you wish you could share with that child or young adult if you had the opportunity?

Parenting is an incredibly stressful and difficult full-time job. Burnout rates are high among teachers, healers, and other helping professionals, particularly those who work in challenging environments with suffering children who are physically or emotionally ill. Too often these places are understaffed, the jobs are underpaid, and the people in them are burned out and stressed. This is why mindfulness practices are so important for you, the adult, to practice as well as teach. Mindfulness practice can help restore the compassion and hope that first brought us to parenting or to work with children. It can repair, nurture, and sustain our idealism.

Practicing what you teach is also critical because kids, adolescents in particular, can spot a phony from a mile away. Your children and the children you work with can sense if you're familiar with the challenges of meditation. When you practice with your children, you experience the challenges and rewards together.

When we first begin meditation, we may think of all the other things we could, or believe we should, be doing, and feel more stressed than ever. The task is to simply notice these feelings of guilt or stress, nervousness, and longing, label them, and let them pass. One of the biggest expectations—and misconceptions—of meditation is that it will be about blissfully experiencing nothing; the reality is that it is about experiencing everything both outside and inside of ourselves, the pleasant as well as the unpleasant.

Basic Meditation Practices for Children and Adults

The Buddha passed through a small village once, where simple farmers lived. One of them approached and asked him, "What do you do all day?" "It's simple," the Buddha replied. "We sit, we walk, and we eat." "That's what we do every day," responded the peasant. "What makes you so special?" "When we sit, we know we are sitting. When we walk, we know we are walking. When we eat, we know we are eating," the Buddha replied.

* *Practice 2.1: Sitting and Lying Down Meditation*

Begin by setting an intention for yourself to have an open mind and to try your best to be patient with yourself. Find a comfortable, quiet spot, inside or outside, where you know you can be free of external distractions for a while. For sitting meditation, you can sit on a chair, a meditation cushion, or a bench, whichever is most comfortable for your body. You can also kneel or have your back supported by a wall or chair if that is more comfortable. The more comfortable you are, the longer you will be able to sit.

Relax as fully as you can, spine and neck straight but not rigid, with your chin comfortable and slightly in and down. Feel as if your spine is coming out of strong roots in the earth and your heart is open to the sky. Don't be afraid to move around a little until you find a comfortable balance. Notice the sensations and thoughts that arise with each shift.

Notice your contact points with the ground and the cushion or chair, and allow your body and the seat to hold you. Imagine yourself sitting like a puppet: a string from the center of your head lifts your spine and head straight, while gravity does the rest of the work of keeping you balanced.

For a lying down meditation, simply lie comfortably on your

back with your arms next to you, your palms facing upward, letting the ground hold you and allowing your body to relax. Your feet should be about hip width apart, and will probably naturally fall to the side.

Relax the muscles in your face and then in the rest of your body. You can clench all your muscles and then let go to help them relax. Rest your eyes gently on the floor about three feet in front of you if you are sitting. You may feel more comfortable with your eyes closed. If you find yourself to be drowsy, open your eyes a bit; if you find your mind distracted by things in the room, close your eyes gently. Breathe in through your nose. This will prevent your mouth from becoming too dry. Quickly scan your body again, noting any tension and letting it go.

Once you are sitting or lying in a meditation position, slowly bring your attention to your breath. Just observe your breathing without trying to change it. Your body will breathe for you. Observe the different physical aspects of breathing, the rise and fall of your belly, the cool air against your nostrils on the in-breath, and the warm air leaving your body on the out-breath. Wherever you most notice your breath, maintain your attention there, simply watching the breath as it rises and falls.

Feel your breathing in your belly. If you like, place one hand on your belly and one on your chest. Breathing from the chest is a sign of stress, and lowers your oxygen intake to less than what your body needs to function optimally and remain relaxed. Try to shift the breath downward into the belly and resume focusing on the breath there.

Each time your mind wanders, gently return your attention to your breathing. You probably won't have to wait long before the mind wanders again. This time, as your mind wanders, try to observe where it's going without going along for the ride. Return to observing your breath, knowing that you are breathing. Notice the different qualities of the breath; some breaths will be smooth, some are long, some short. Note anything that arises, each time naming the thought or feeling and then coming back to the breath.

———— *

One of the most difficult parts of this practice is cultivating patience and self-compassion. What you are experiencing is the perfectly natural and expected "monkey mind" that will wander off in search of bananas or whatever else happens to be floating down the stream. I had a meditation teacher say that the mind secretes thought just as the pancreas secretes insulin, and we have about as much luck stopping the mind as we do the pancreas. Eventually, the mind, like a small puppy, will begin to settle and remain in place for longer periods of time. You are building your concentration muscle. To begin, just enjoy watching your mind as you would a new puppy. Where does he go? Does she run to the future, the past, worried places, or excited places? Simply observe the thoughts, feelings, and physical sensations. Label them and return your attention to the breath. Remember to stop, observe, and return, and try not to judge yourself or your thoughts. That stopping and returning creates concentration and calm. Observation and nonjudgment strengthen our wisdom, insight, and compassion.

As you become accustomed to relaxing with the chaos of your mind during meditation, you'll become more relaxed when outer chaos swirls around you. Trust that if those urgent thoughts are important enough, they will come back to you later. Trying to forcibly stop your thoughts won't work. Only by calmly observing them do you allow them to settle.

You may want to quit sitting right away. Don't get mad at your urge to quit, but don't quit either. You may have urges to move—try to notice them and not give in. If you do adjust or scratch a mosquito bite, do it mindfully. Be aware of what you are doing, the urge, the movement of your muscles, and the relief…as well as the inevitable return of the itch.

Start with a five-minute sitting period. At some point, you may choose to sit for longer periods of time. A sitting meditation period in a practice center is often twenty to twenty-five minutes or longer, but remember that at any point in the day, you can always re-center and check in with your breath in less than a minute.

Insight meditation teacher Jack Kornfield often tells this story about focusing on the breath. A novice monk in a monastery was meditating by a stream and finding himself growing bored with simply focusing on the breath all day. The master approached and asked him how he was doing. "I'm just so sick and tired of focusing on the breath.

It's boring!" he complained. The master paused for a moment, then suddenly and without warning thrust the head of the novice monk into the stream. The novice struggled and gasped, choking and trying to get his head above water, but the master held him down as he splashed and panicked. Finally the master let go. "Master, why did you do this to me?" cried the monk. "I wanted to ask you," replied the master, "is the breath interesting now?"

The breath may be more interesting to us at some points than at others, but it is always available—anywhere, anytime—it's nicely portable. As the joke goes, "If you aren't able to breathe, then you've definitely got more important things to worry about." If you find you need a regular reminder to focus on your breathing, you can count your breaths, counting "one" for the first in- and out-breath, "two" for the second, and so on up to ten and then starting over again with one. You can also try adding words that narrate your experience, for example: "Breathing in happiness, breathing out sadness; breathing in acceptance, breathing out anger; breathing in patience, breathing out frustration; breathing in gratitude, breathing out selfishness."

Daily Life Mindfulness Meditations

We don't need to stop and sit in a particular posture to practice mindfulness meditation. Here's a simple water-drinking meditation that creates awareness of the mind, the body, and our impulses. It can be done with the first few sips of water you take with a meal. You can also try this with other favorite drinks: milk, tea, lemonade, or juice.

* *Practice: 2.2: Mindful Water Drinking*[13]

Pour yourself a cool glass of water. Look at it, and consider where it comes from, tracing it back through the faucet or the factory to a natural water source, from the sky and beyond. Notice any bubbles, or the way the water refracts the light. Now take a small sip of the water. Allow it to rest on your tongue and flow in your mouth, noticing how your mouth naturally responds. Notice the sensations, the flavors, and the feelings of relief or pleasure that may accompany drinking. As you swallow, notice your muscles contracting, the sensations and sounds in your throat and the response of your belly. What is happening in the mind, thoughts, emotions? Do you find you desire more? Is your hand already moving to lift the glass up? Try a few more sips this way. Try gulping the water and noting the varying responses your mind and body have.

If you do this meditation regularly at different times of day, you will begin to notice different responses. Sometimes you will be thirsty, sated, warm, cold, or in various other emotional and physical states. If you do it with the first sips of water of every glass, it gets to be a habit and easy to remember.

Metta Meditation

We all have moments when we go into a situation trying not to be present or wishing we were somewhere else. As a teacher and therapist, I have had mornings when I wanted to avoid the entire day of work after thinking about having to interact with that one difficult child or co-worker. This is hardly staying present in the moment, this is getting paralyzed by a future that may or may not even happen! Metta is a loving kindness meditation used to help us bring compassion to our colleagues, our adversaries, the world, and ourselves.

Practice 2.3: Metta Meditation[14]

Assume a comfortable sitting meditation position. Gently close your eyes and let yourself relax. Notice your points of contact with the chair and ground, and gradually bring your attention to your breath. When you feel comfortable, place a hand over your heart. After a few breaths, bring to mind a person or "benefactor" who represents pure loving kindness and generosity of spirit to you. Ideally, this is an important person from your childhood—perhaps a patient teacher, counselor, relative, or friend. Maybe it was someone who reached out and showed you compassion when you were struggling, or maybe someone who taught you the value of patience. You could even choose a child who has been important in teaching you, perhaps a student or your own child or a close relative. Imagine this person's presence, how you feel when you're with them, feeling their compassion and generosity. Slowly begin sending them gratitude and wishes for their well-being with this phrase: "May you find happiness, may you find peace, may you live in love and compassion." There are many variations on this phrase; pick one that works for you. Practice this for a few minutes each day.

After a few days of practice, add in a good, trustworthy childhood friend to your imagining. Perhaps it is someone you are still in touch with, or parted ways with, but it should be someone towards whom you have no ill will towards. Imagine their presence and send them the same hopes and good will. Try this for a few days, and then add someone about whom you feel neutral. After a few days of this, try to send the metta wishes to someone who is challenging for you. This could be a colleague, your own child or family member, or a student or client who has been frustrating. This will likely be challenging, but try to stick with it. One helpful way to find compassion for others is to imagine them as children—thinking about their fears and hopes and dreams.

This exercise can be very useful for dealing with strong emotions about challenging children or adults. With some maturity, children can practice metta as well, for the bullies or the frightening adults in their lives. If you're working with young people who have little experience of a positive teacher or benefactor, encourage them to just imagine the presence of someone they feel safe around, even a pet or a favorite fictional character.

At the end of a teen retreat, some older teens and I joked at first and then started talking more seriously about the fun of "stealth metta"—walking around the school sending metta phrases to people in the hallway, or sitting on the subway sending metta to strangers, or anywhere that there are people or living creatures around us. I was listening to a Dharma talk by Narayan Liebensen Grady at the Cambridge Insight Meditation Society when a siren went by one day. She suggested that we say a little metta for whoever was involved in that situation, which is a wonderful way to handle such disruptions when meditating in an urban environment.

I do know that for myself metta practice has helped with my burnout, which usually begins when I start feeling frustrated with other people. I worked at schools in inner-city Boston for many years. Sadly, it was often hard to tell whether the students or staff were more miserable. Everyone slouched around the drab hallways, constantly on edge, and the hopelessness was often palpable and, sadly, contagious. Most teachers ignored my presence and that of my fellow therapists; others were even less friendly to us and downright rude to the children.

One teacher in particular, Ms. F., seemed unnecessarily harsh and very nasty toward the students, snapping at them in the hallway as I walked past with them, or even making remarks to me directly that I was unable to "keep them in line." She would lord it over her corner of the school, looking up from her crossword puzzles only to criticize. It was easy enough to complain about what a lousy teacher she was to my co-workers and bosses. But my supervisor had a different take on the situation. First he pointed out that she was only as toxic as we allowed her to be to each of us as individuals. And he also said, "Try to imagine not that you are treating just the kids, but the whole system: the school, the teachers, the families, and our community." It was a helpful way to reframe, but still felt impractical until a meditation teacher suggested metta.

I had no interest in sending love and compassion to Ms. F., and it took a long time to work my way up to her. But I used, as my neutral people, some of the staff in the school whom I didn't really know, and soon the school started to seem like a friendlier place. I could see the exhaustion and fear in people's faces, whereas before I had only seen anger. With Ms. F., I didn't see a lot of change in her behavior, but I did see a change in my own reactions to her, and in the fact that I often started reacting before I'd even seen her. I tried to visualize what she might have been like as a child and young adult, and what her life may have been like and why she went into working with kids. We certainly didn't become friends. I didn't interact much more with her, but I no longer let her keep me in bed in the morning dreading going in to work and facing an interaction with her. Just that shift made my whole experience of the work environment different, and I could feel my stress fading.

✻ *Practice 2.4: Attunement*

Another way to practice mindfulness when your child or someone around you is particularly challenging is attunement, aligning with a child, a client, or a colleague's emotional and spiritual state. There are a few ways to do this. One is to try subtly mirroring the person's body language, making sure you are not exaggerating or "mocking" their movements. Another is to simply visualize a connection between your two hearts as you sit across from each other or even side-by-side. Another tip I got from an acupuncturist that I found particularly helpful is to slowly align my breath with that of the person I am working with, feeling their level of anxiety and then gradually bringing both of our breaths down to a more relaxed pace. This creates an unconscious bond of safety and connection that allows for more trust to flow back and forth between two people. I've often experienced children whose strong emotion is escalating calming down just by having someone sit next to them without saying anything and aligning their breath and body language.

✻

✻ *Practice 2.5: Mindfulness Bells*

In the chaos of even an ordinary day, it is helpful to have some visual or auditory reminder to return us to mindfulness. On retreats, Thich Nhat Hanh rings a mindfulness bell at random times throughout the day, during which the retreatants stop, pause, and focus on the present moment. We too can find and create "mindfulness bells" sprinkled throughout our day. These bells do not need to be actual bells, but anything that happens—sounds or events—throughout our days. Some ideas of possible mindfulness bells include:

* Red lights or stop signs
* Waiting for your computer to boot up when you get to work
* The ringing of a telephone
* A staircase
* A doorknob
* Waiting for a pot to boil or coffee to brew
* A subway train pulling into a station
* Picking up an object (e.g., toothbrush, coffee mug)
* Standing in line
* Waiting for your bread to toast or your food to heat up
* Turning on the faucet
* Waiting a few breaths before checking your text messages or email

Each time you encounter a bell, remember to stop, observe, and return to the present moment. Simply quiet yourself, observe what is happening inside and outside, and take three mindful breaths before returning to what you were doing.

A mindfulness bell works best when it is connected to activities that you are already doing. A teacher once suggested to me driving one leg of my commute once a week without listening to the radio or talking on the phone or drinking my coffee. I didn't think much of the idea at first, but when I tried it and I felt the vibrations of the car, the sounds of the engine that reminded me to shift, I was much more aware of the thoughts and feelings that arose as I cut even one distraction out of a regular activity. Even the first and last five minutes of a drive in silence helps ease my transition to the next space.

Another mindfulness bell is to commit to noticing one beautiful thing each day, perhaps on your commute. It could be a tree beginning to blossom, a particularly beautiful shaft of light, even a house painted in one of your favorite colors. Start a list of these beautiful things in your journal or share it with friends on an email thread to remind each other of the beauty in the world.

You may also keep an actual bell in your home, office, or classroom to ring at times throughout the day, a common practice on retreats. If you work at a desk and computer, you can download a mindfulness bell tone that will ring a few times throughout the day, bringing you back to the present moment. You can even photocopy pictures of a bell and post them around a school, or get cards or stickers printed and laminated to hand out or carry in your pocket or wallet.

Some families use the bell as a way to bring the family together before eating. Even young children can learn to sit quietly with their breath for the length of the sound of the bell or to take three breaths whenever they hear it.

Expanding Outward and Sustaining your Practice

Once you have been meditating or practicing mindfulness for a while, it will become clear that although meditation or mindfulness may be simple enough for a child to grasp or even do, it hardly remains easy. One of the more challenging parts of practice is simply finding the time. Schedule a regular time of day that you look forward to, rather than making meditation an obligation you are trying to squeeze into your busy day. Consistent practice is important; practicing meditation is like exercising a muscle. You have to do it regularly to keep it in shape and it may take time to see the benefits. You are probably not in shape after eating and sleeping through the holidays, even if you played soccer all Fall. Find a time early in the morning, or perhaps right after work or exercise, that you can commit to each day. Tie it to something else in your day that is already a part of your routine, like after you shower or while you are waiting for your coffee to brew.

After a time, you can integrate mindfulness into more of your daily activities. One of the most sustaining ways to practice is with someone else or with a group or community, sometimes called a "Sangha." Each child and adult can help support the community in sitting quietly, drinking mindfully, or remembering a mindfulness bell. If you are using these practices alone or with your clients or students, it's nourishing to find a group, another teacher, parent, or colleague who you can practice with and support. Even just one other person who is practicing with you or supporting your practice will encourage you to practice more; you and one grandchild or patient are enough to make a community that supports practice. I even know of groups of friends emerging from retreats who set their watches to take a mindful moment at the same time of day, joining together in reflection and awareness in spite of their physical distance, miles and even continents apart.

Your Sangha can be a meditation or spiritual center, it can be your workplace, your family, or your partner. Experts on behavioral change also recommend committing yourself to something publicly—so even if you don't have a meditation community, tell people you are going to start practicing regularly. With time, they may want to join you.

Over time, if you stick with meditation, you will naturally find new ways to relax. You may find yourself slowing down and enjoying your meal. Perhaps you will become aware that you are listening more deeply to others in conversations rather than merely waiting to speak; maybe you are not so frustrated when driving in traffic. You may realize that you are taking better care of yourself, listening to your body's needs and responding appropriately. Your mind will take care of your body, and your body will reciprocate. Where you were once in the habit of seeking fleeting relief, you may now be engaged in activities that create longer-term happiness in yourself and in those around you.

With some practice and time studying your mind through meditation, you will probably start to notice patterns in your thoughts. You will inevitably re-encounter the same storylines over and over. Some of these will be pleasant, some not so pleasant, but notice how your mind and body's responses change depending on your mood, your body, and other factors. Where do these stories come from? Whose voices are they? How long have you been listening to them? Try to observe them, remembering they are mere mental creations that may or may not reflect reality. You don't have to believe everything you think. Watch them like leaves floating down a stream, don't jump in the river and chase them, just watch them drifting by. Shift your usual perspective and intend to look *at* the thoughts, not from them.[15] What is the shape of thought, the physical sensation? Does the mind interpret events and respond before your consciousness sets to work? As Nietzsche once said, "There are no facts, only interpretations."

3

Practicing with Children

When I was a boy of 14, my father was so ignorant I could hardly stand to have the old man around. But when I got to be 21, I was astonished at how much the old man had learned in seven years.
—Mark Twain

When I transitioned from working as a psychotherapist with adults to working with children, I was astonished by their open-mindedness and the intensity of their curiosity. Spending time with young people is a gift in that we see the world through the fresh eyes of a child—mindfully. Even adolescents I worked with, once I got past their too-cool veneer, would quickly become engaged and excited. Young people are so often the living embodiment of the Zen "beginner's mind." Young people seem to respond to meditation out of this natural inquisitiveness. Sadly, as they grow older, our culture pushes this innate curiosity aside in favor of productivity, conformity, and consumption. But we can still offer meditation as a powerful and lifelong gift, in a way that nurtures this innate interest and allows it to thrive in our culture.

Even if your children are initially resistant or skeptical about mindfulness practices, don't give up. Your goal is to "plant the seeds of mindfulness," as Thich Nhat Hanh says, and offer the possibility of the meditation practice as a helpful and playful tool. I worked with one young man who, through some poor choices, was facing many years in prison. While there, he was able to access meditation practices that had been taught to him when he was younger. The practice brought relief to his suffering and eventually he became a resource and teacher for those around him.

When teaching mindfulness to children, I start by remembering Chogyam Trungpa's Six Points of Mindful Speech, summarized here.

Practice 3.1 Six Points of Mindful Speech

1. Pay attention to your own speech, not just to what you are saying, but how you talk. Really listen to yourself talking.
2. Listen to other people and how they speak, particularly children or teens. The focus is not primarily on the content, but the point is to pay attention to *how* people talk.
3. Enunciate clearly.
4. Slow down your speech slightly, so that you pay more attention and put more emphasis on individual words.
5. Simplify your speech. You don't have to use as many words or talk as much as you think you do, especially with children.
6. Pay attention to the space around the word, not just the words themselves, but the rhythm and silences of speech.

The practices in this book are multisensory, borrowing from various cultures and incorporating games, art, and stories to assist children's learning. For the sake of organization, some exercises have been linked to certain chapters and topics. I want to be clear that all of these exercises will be helpful for any child, teen, or even adult.

Be direct with the children in your life about why you think they would benefit from mindfulness meditation. Consider what specific goals they may have or changes they would like to make. These may include relaxation, better sleep, a way to deal with boredom or with the frustration over everyday events, better academic or athletic performance, improved memory and creativity, and less suffering from physical or emotional pain.

In my experience, most kids, particularly younger and more troubled kids, do not respond all that well to explicit suggestions about what needs changing. This is not unlike the challenge of getting some children to eat broccoli; no matter how delicious you make it, once you tell them it's good for them, that fork goes down. Instead, make these meditative activities pleasant by associating them with pleasant feelings or fun activities. If we offer to show children a magic trick about their ears and walk them through a few sound-counting exercises, the child may first respond with a sigh and eye roll at the worst, but by the end they are often impressed and come to wonder at the mystery of how much had gone unnoticed before. Jokingly asking a child if they know how to breathe, which can be a good route to introducing mindful breathing exercises. Telling a story about where food comes from or letting your child in on the "secret" of discovering a seed in the raisin during a mindful eating activity is much better received than saying, "You need to learn to eat more mindfully." Align the effects of mindfulness with the child's goals and interests, not just your own. For example, "This type of breathing is used by famous athletes and coaches to help their game, and by famous performers to keep calm during concerts in front of thousands." Make it useful; for example, "This is a little trick to keep you from getting bored while you're waiting in line."

Linking activities with the right role model or an aspect of pop culture can be very powerful, something advertisers know well. Of course, navigate the treacherous waters of what's cool and what isn't in today's pop culture at your own peril. Generally speaking, ninja, athletes, and samurai will probably remain eternally cool to kids. *Star Wars* references, specific athletes, and music groups like the Wu-Tang Clan or the Beastie Boys may or may not already be outdated.

Often when I have introduced meditation to kids as a solution to a problem they would rather forget, the child tends to shut down because I have reminded her of the problem. For example, if I say, "I've got this activity that will help you with your ADHD," the child hears "ADHD" and is reminded about what makes her different and ostracized by peers. The purpose of mindfulness is not to fix something that is broken, but rather to build on existing strengths.

Remember also that what we adults think of as fun and relaxing, like playing an instrument or reading a book, may feel like a chore to kids. "Go practice your meditation" should never, ever feel required. Finally, just as meditation should not become associated with a punishment, meditation should never, ever, become a chore. Remember that as soon as we make anything a chore, or even too important to adults, we start shutting down that natural curiosity and playfulness. When you practice, you begin to see what the challenges and rewards are over time—just like going to work or to the gym.

Short Introductory Mindfulness Activities

Visual, physical, and hands-on demonstrations are often more powerful than simple verbal explanations. Using tasks like washing chalkboards to demonstrate that we need to clear the mind of the day's residue is a good example, especially when old chalk marks are still visible beneath the erasing. Snow globes make excellent visual demonstrations of settling the whirlwind of the mind and its swirling thoughts that need to settle, and of course, the harder we try to make it settle, the less it does. Glitter balls and wands also work well for this. The children's mindfulness teacher Kimberly Post Rowe recommends demonstrating mind-body connections, like taking a child's pulse or temperature before and after a meditation activity. She also suggests having children close their eyes and simply visualize biting into a lemon. They will be amazed to notice that their face and tongue have reacted to the sour taste, just from imagining it. Some children also find themselves unconsciously making a fist when they think about becoming angry, or even becoming angry when they make a fist.

Setting Expectations

If you are trying these practices one-on-one, it might not be necessary to set up a formal time when you teach mindfulness, but if you are in a group or a large family setting, establishing basic expectations is essential. It's no fun, or even effective, to get bogged down with too many rules. Rather, if you don't already have these expectations in your family or classroom, ask everyone in the group to agree on certain expectations. For example, can everyone agree to be as quiet as possible? Can everyone agree to raise hands if they have a question? Older children might be able to come up with expectations themselves. For discussions in bigger groups, you might wish to pass a talking stick or stone that is then held by the person who is speaking and passed to the next speaker.

Where to Create Your Meditation Space

In theory, mindfulness can be practiced anywhere. However, especially when you are beginning practicing mindfulness with your children, designating a space reserved specifically for meditation and free of other distractions can be really helpful. The space itself, a dedicated room or even a corner, can serve as a reminder to come back to ourselves each time we walk by. Even a classroom can have a quiet meditation corner, and it needn't be perfect; the purpose is to cultivate a calm space inside of ourselves, not the perfect space around us.

If you're working with a group, mindfully creating a meditation space together can be an excellent initial group activity. You may want to make a nondenominational altar and decorate it with objects that are meaningful to you and the children. Bring some of your own special items and encourage the children to bring in objects or mementos that are special to them, and whose beauty or meaning they want to share. Objects can be collected on a mindful walk outside, where people can pick up beautiful stones, flowers, feathers, and other things. Include items in the space that represent the six senses: sight, touch, sound, taste, smell, and thought. Bring soft fabrics or smooth stones for touch, perhaps some citrus fruits or pine needles for smell, something to represent taste, a bell or music for sound. The space should be as quiet and free of distractions as possible, away from sounds like television or over-stimulating views—for example, near the playground. If you have access to a calm outdoor space, by all means make use of it.

When to Introduce Mindfulness Practice

While mindfulness can be incorporated throughout the day, when starting out it's helpful to have a consistent time and place to practice mindfulness meditations. Parents may want to introduce regular moments throughout the day, just before dinner or early in the morning for the family to take a few mindful breaths together. Teachers may find it useful to create a routine at the beginning or end of class, and therapists and doctors may want to use the start and end of meetings. A great time is after returning from gym or recess. Routines can incorporate sensory cues, so that children become habituated to meditation time. These might include dimming the lights, inviting the bell to sound, playing soft music, or other cues that will come to be associated with meditation time. Such routines can help children settle and get used to these unfamiliar activities. Once practices become routine, children are better able to internalize the values and effects. I think daily regularity for even a few moments is probably better than a long stretch of practice time once a week.

Creating a regular time helps you as the adult from turning mindfulness into a punishment or "time out." Teach and reinforce the skills and activities regularly when the child is in a good mood with an open mind and heart. Let him or her learn in these moments in order to reap the benefits for helping with later, difficult times.

Of course, difficult times inevitably arise like violent storms, and it becomes tempting to remind an actively suffering or raging child that they have meditation as a tool. There are skillful and unskillful ways to help a child access their mindfulness. If we always remind him or her in response to a bad behavior, meditation may come to be associated with punishment. Instead, with regular practice, kids are more likely to avoid getting into a tantrum situation in the first place. Trust that if a child can learn in a safe place, he or she will eventually remember in a crisis. Practice in good times increases the likelihood of mindful awareness in the times it is needed most. Athletes don't train just the day of the competition, but they practice and work out for months or years before the big day.

Helping Children in Difficult Moments

Of course, we do want to help children when they're in a purely emotional state, whether they are experiencing anger, anxiety, or sadness, and this can be quite a challenge. It's not so easy to talk a frustrated child into taking a few deep breaths or counting to ten, even if we know such a practice would be helpful. Telling a child in the midst of a tantrum, "You're too angry, go to your room and practice breathing!"

is not likely to help. I have witnessed frustrated adults screaming at children, "Calm down, just take a deep breath and count to ten!" I'm still waiting to see this work effectively.

This is why cultivating mindful awareness and stillness in ourselves is so crucial. When we find ourselves in those tense situations, it can be hard not to take our child's anger or fear or frustration into ourselves; emotions, particularly strong emotions, are contagious—even research shows this. It's upsetting to watch someone be upset, especially if we feel powerless to make it better, and our own hearts and minds are probably closed if we too are overwhelmed. This is the perfect time, as the adult, to mirror mindfulness practice. If you're upset, the child is probably upset, and suggest practicing together rather than demanding that the child comply or breathe. You can say, "You know what, I think we're both feeling upset, why don't we take a few deep breaths together." or "Wow, I'm feeling really frustrated. Sometimes it calms me down to count ten breaths. Since we got mad together, maybe we can calm down together."

These thoughtful, relational responses are more effective than merely telling a child to count to ten or to practice breathing. When we practice with a child, we learn from and become role models for each other.

I was recently at a conference where I heard about a study of restraints in residential facilities. After examining a number of factors in the children and in the institutions, they found that the staff personalities and stress levels were often the most important variable in how many restraints were used with residents. More than any other variable, a calm staff led to calm residents. Certain staff, those who were able to maintain their calm, were able to calmly de-escalate the children verbally before anything approached an actual hands-on restraint. This is a powerful argument for good staff training, especially mindfulness training for staff in inpatient and high-risk settings. Sometimes, compassionate presence is the best thing we can cultivate in ourselves; the Dalai Lama has been quoted as saying, "We can live without religion and meditation, but we cannot survive without human affection."[16] The more we teach our children affection and compassion directly and through modeling, the more they too can offer it to each other and build for themselves a more compassionate world.

I've often found dealing with my own ego and expectations a more difficult challenge than dealing with some of the toughest children. I've worked with troubled children for a long time, and when I started out I had high expectations of the power of mindfulness—well, my mindfulness. I imagined my chaotic classroom at the mental hospital suddenly transformed into an oasis of peace. In the fantasy, not only did the kids come to practice mindfulness on their own—their emotional and behavioral issues cured—but the other teachers and staff sought out my wisdom in classroom management and clinical theories. This hardly happened, but once I let go of the struggle, I came to appreciate the occasional moments of peace that did come a bit more often with patience and practice.

I sometimes encounter people who have come out the other side. I worked with a man who had recently been released from prison. He remembered and clearly treasured a time spent with a yoga instructor who had paid a visit to the prison many years before. The man had practiced almost daily since then and was one of the most engaged members of the mindfulness group at the halfway house. Someone had planted the seeds of freedom and taught him to water them.

And if we are planting seeds in a child to blossom in the community, we must tend our entire garden, ourselves, and each other. If you are a parent, practice as a family. Recommend a mindfulness curriculum at school or in your place of worship. Volunteer to come in and lead a meditation. Be part of creating a mindful school community where teachers and students can reinforce each other's contemplative practice. If you're a therapist or doctor, teach the whole family you work with to practice together. The more places that a child is reminded of mindful awareness, the more places the seeds you planted will be nurtured and can thrive.

Intentions and Expectations

It is vital to keep checking in with ourselves and our intentions, as well as our expectations for the children. Ask yourself, What are my goals? Are they reasonable given the child I am working with? Have I become too attached to the idea of this child changing or learning to meditate? Have I become too attached to my role as a teacher? And no matter how important meditation or mindfulness practice may be to you personally, it may not be the right time for the child you are trying to teach. Pema Chodron writes, "The truth you believe and cling to makes you unavailable to hear anything new," and often we blind ourselves by clinging to the idea that meditation is the one answer. Remain aware of your own hopes but beware of attachment to outcomes. Realistic expectations are very different from low expectations, and hopes should not be confused with expectations. This practice is challenging for lifelong practitioners, so it will certainly be difficult for children. But remember too that frustration and failure have often been the best teachers of the masters.

If you work with young people, you probably know that patience and a good sense of humor are two of your best tools. Teaching adults to meditate takes enormous reserves of these, and teaching children takes even more. Take the children seriously, but don't take yourself too seriously. Do not be afraid to have a sense of humor about yourself and even your students in a respectful way; it's a great way to model acceptance and how to handle frustration, and to show that meditation and life are fun. If humor isn't your strength, you can work on it, but more importantly, work on your strength—whether that is the arts or language or just your own compassionate presence.

The ancient teachers remind us to sit in meditation with no hope of fruition. Teach with no such hope either, but teach with the right intention. Teach from the heart because you believe this can help or heal, not because you have expectations or attachments to outcomes.

Oh, and have fun.

✻ *Practice 3.2 Tips to Teach By*

- Create as quiet and comfortable a space as possible.
- Introduce the activity, setting clear expectations.
- Remain aware of your own intentions and goals before and during teaching, letting go of expectations.
- Smile and breathe.
- Speak in a calm but strong voice, remaining aware of your nonverbal communication.
- Consider age-appropriate language and metaphor.
- Remain connected, trusting, empathic, and nonjudgmental of yourself and your children.

* Keep your sense of humor and patience.
* Have at least a Plan B.
* Cultivate curiosity and creativity .
* Start small and build up.
* Stay positive, engage the positive.
* Practice and encourage practice whenever possible.
* Take your work seriously, but don't take yourself seriously.

Mindfulness Practices

4

Core Mindfulness Practices for Children

It is easier to build strong children than to repair broken men.
—Frederick Douglass

The first meditation I ever learned was a gift from my father, when I was probably about six years old. We were floating on a raft in a pond and gazing up at the blue summer sky. Above us we watched as giant cumulus clouds slowly morphed into new forms and then gradually un-formed. My dad looked over at me and said, "Hey, want to see a magic trick?" Of course I did. "I'm going to make a cloud disappear with my mind." "No way!" I responded. "Sure, I'll do it. In fact, we can do it together. Pick a cloud, let's start with a small one to practice." I picked a smallish looking puffy white cloud just visible on the horizon. "Now, all you have to do is focus on that cloud and just breathe. With each breath, notice the cloud getting a little bit smaller." We lay there in the sun looking at the cloud, breathing together and sure enough, with each breath the cloud seemed to fade slightly. "Keep focusing on that cloud," my father instructed me. "Bring your mind back if it wanders; you have to keep your mind on it or it won't disappear." We continued breathing, focusing, and sending our will to the cloud as it faded away over the course of the next few minutes. It was certainly magic to me. Of course, now I understand that clouds will form and un-form in the sky regardless of my intention and willpower. But still, at that moment, my breath and my mind seemed like the most powerful forces in the world. Second only, maybe, to my Dad.

Try this meditation yourself first to get a sense of the best clouds; it really only works with the puffy white cumulous ones. You can even try placing your worries onto the cloud, and letting them fade slowly away. But once you get the hang of it, pass it on to a child as my father did to me.

✻ *Practice 4.1: Cloud Concentration Meditation*

Pick out a cloud; you may want to start with a small one. Focus on that cloud and just breathe into the cloud. With each breath, watch and see if that cloud changes shape or starts to get smaller. If your mind wanders, which it might, just notice that and bring your attention and breath back to the cloud. Just remain focused on the cloud, watching and breathing, until it gradually fades away.

✻

The forming and un-forming, ever-changing nature of the clouds is a great first lesson for children in the power of the breath. It is also a wonderful reminder that everything from the most intense feeling to the puffiest cloud will inevitably change and ultimately fade.

Eating Meditations

This next meditation can be done with an orange or clementine or other sweet citrus fruit. Oranges make for great eating meditation as they stimulate all the senses with their bumpy outer peel and inner stickiness, bright color, bright powerful scent, and sweet flavor. Even the sound of the peel tearing off can be surprisingly evocative. In this exercise, children truly get to know an orange.

✻ *Practice 4.2: Know Your Orange*[17]

This practice works well for a group and also one-on-one. Seat the group around a basket of oranges or clementines. Ask the child or children if they can tell them apart. Then have every member of the group come and select an orange. Then ask them the following questions. Feel free to add others. How many colors do you see when you look closely? What shape is your orange? What else is on the orange? Where do you think it was before it was in this basket, this house, this building?

Ask the children to close their eyes and notice what it feels like. Ask these questions: What does your orange feel like when you squeeze it in different places, how does the peel feel against your skin, your hand, your face? Bringing the orange to your nose, can you smell anything special? How far from your nose can you smell the orange? What is special and unique about your orange?

Collect the oranges from the group and return them to the table. Now you can invite the children up one at a time to find their orange (you might want to consider an order to make this easier for some children). Once everyone has found their orange, enjoy eating the fruits of your labor. This time, remember to keep your nose open as you peel, listen carefully to the sounds, and enjoy fully tasting each juicy, sweet segment.

✻

While all the sense meditations can be used to talk about our human interconnection to the different parts of the universe, this works particularly well with eating meditation. For the exercise below, I use raisins because they're small, not messy, and easy to pass out to a group of children, but any other food would work as well.

✻ *Practice 4.3: The Universe in a Raisin*

Hold up a raisin and ask your child or children where it comes from. Trace all the human elements that have interacted with the raisin, such as the person who planted the grape vine, harvested the grapes, dried them, and brought them to market. It may help to write or chart them out on a piece of paper or chalkboard. Don't forget everyone from yourself to the checkout person, the person who stocks the shelves, the truck driver, the truck loader, the packer, the factory worker, the driver from the farm, and the gas-station attendant. Consider too the families and friends of those people, the people who gave birth to them and raised them, the people who built the truck and tilled the soil. Have each child present pick a figure from the raisin's story and draw a picture or write a short story about that person's contribution to the raisin. Read back the story or look at the pictures before slowly and mindfully eating the raisin.

This exercise works really well across the age spectrum. Young children are able to get interested in the idea of how many people have touched their tiny raisin, and older children and teenagers can get the sense of how much is involved in what they consume. This is also a powerful exercise for adults. My friend Ryan, who has been in recovery from drug addiction for many years, told me recently that a major factor in his decision to get sober came after he was exposed to the idea of mindful consumption when he saw all the suffering, exploitation, and violence associated with the drug trade that he was part of. This shook his awareness when he realized he wasn't only harming himself and perhaps a few people close to him, but rather he was part of a system that was creating suffering in communities across the globe.

Another interconnectedness exercise is to trace all the ingredients of the raisin and where they came from. Begin by explaining that the raisin is a cloud or a star, and trace this back to the grape on the vine, back to the dirt in the ground that came from other composted plants, the water that came from the hose, that came from the reservoir, that came from the clouds above, that could have come from an ocean thousands of miles away that was warmed by the star that is our sun, and remember the sunshine that gave the grapes the energy to grow. When you eat your raisin, you eat the entire universe. When you interact with anyone or anything, you've interacted with everyone and everything. This is a thought-provoking and truly perspective-changing exercise. Introducing this awareness also lays the groundwork for a larger project like cleaning up an old lot, composting for a garden, planting vegetables, cooking them, and then composting the leftovers again.

Another sensory meditation focuses specifically on smell.

✻ *Practice 4.4: What the Nose Knows*[18]

Find a few objects with powerful and evocative odors. Some ideas include a citrus peel, a cinnamon stick, fresh ginger, chocolate, herbs or spices, tea leaves, or even non-food items like flowers, pine needles, grass, or soil—anything that can bring up powerful memories and associations. Have the children sit mindfully breathing in a circle with eyes closed, and hand them the object. Have the children breathe out and raise the object to their nose, then inhale deeply. Let them do this quietly for a few breaths and then ask the following questions: What thoughts begin to emerge? Do you want more of this smell or less? Does the smell make you remember anything? Have you smelled it before? Where exactly in your nose or mouth do you notice the smell or taste? Does it remind you of any particular people, places, or times? What thoughts or feelings come up with those memories? Does your stomach growl, your mouth water, or your nose wrinkle without your mind even asking it to?

Invite the children to discuss the experience of what came up in their minds for them, based just on a simple odor. Writing or drawing about the experience or thoughts that arose makes for a fun creative writing or art project.

✻

✻ *Practice 4.5: Mindfulness of Touch*[19]

This fun children's game is really a lesson in mindfulness of touch. It works best in a group setting but can be adapted for a smaller family practice. Have the children sit mindfully in a circle with hands behind their back. Place an object in each child's hands without showing the child or the others. Now that they have the object, they have to try to figure out what it is. Children take turns explaining to the group what they think they are holding. Talk about shape, texture, size, and other qualities. Fun objects can include dice, game pieces, coins, marbles, shells, pinecones, toys, a marker or crayon, small statues, or other souvenirs. Go around the circle until each child has had a turn. Discuss how much we can learn from touch if we are paying attention and what we can't learn (such as color and taste) from this one sense, and what kinds of thoughts and feelings arise with being limited in our perceptions.

*

If you are trying these practices with your family, you may want to try this hugging meditation exercise created by Thich Nhat Hanh. He introduces it by saying that the purpose of the hugging meditation is to bring more awareness to your hugging by incorporating mindful breathing and an awareness of the preciousness of the person in your arms. Children could do it at home, first practicing it with family and close friends they hug already. They should always be given the option of not having to do it, and it should only be done with people that the children already hug regularly and are comfortable with.

You can also try this exercise without the physical touching, just practicing being close to each other and looking at each other, if that is more comfortable.

* *Practice 4.6: Hugging Meditation*

Face your partner and look into his or her eyes. Giggling is a fine way to begin.

Smiling, slowly approach each other, taking one mindful step at a time together. Feel the earth below you with each step. Notice any feelings in your body as you get closer to the other person, particularly around your stomach. What does your body or mind want to do? Run toward, run away? Nothing? Now just a half a foot apart, look at each other. You may want to stop here and just practice looking at each other from what feels like a safe distance. What do you feel? What do you think? What do you see in your partner's eyes? Can you notice the rhythm of that person's breath?

If you and your child are comfortable with this, lean in and hug each other. Allow three deep breaths for the hug. Feel the warmth, the other person's heartbeat, notice any thoughts and feelings that arise. Giggling is fine here too. Now take one step back, then another, trying to keep eye contact. You can think something nice for your partner, a wish for them, at this point. Breaking eye contact, look back down, and just focus on your own breath, slowly letting your breath return to its own rhythm. If you have siblings that are close enough to each other, they can try the exercise together as well.

This exercise can lead to rich discussions about our awareness of others, giving and receiving affection, noticing limits of comfort, and recognizing the preciousness of another person alive in your arms.

The Big Om

Rhythmic chanting and music make a wonderful sensory meditation for many children who may not respond as well to verbal or physical activities. This meditation simply repeats the word "om," the original sound of the universe in Hindu belief. The exercise is best done sitting in a circle on the ground, but anywhere will do.

Practice 4.7: The Big Om[20]

This is the script to use with children:

In India and many other places in the world, it is believed that when the universe was born, it let out a great vibration that you can still hear today if you listen carefully, connecting you to the origin of the universe. Perhaps we can think of it as the vibrations of the big bang, or just the hum of the Earth when we are absolutely quiet and still. It sounds like this: Auummmmmmm. (Let out a big one.) Now you try it. (Let the children make their om.) Okay, now we will see how long we can all hold the om together. Auummmmmmmm.

(Wait until all the children have finished and are catching their breath.) Could you feel that? Could you feel the power? This time, we will say the om and just keep going with it. When you run out of air, just breathe and start again, so that the sound is continuous. (While the children are oming, bring in some words of encouragement.) Feel the om coming from deep in your belly, feel the vibration up and down your body, feel the vibration going downward into the earth...and the om of the earth moving into you, feel your own body and power, the vibration in your chest and throat, feel the vibration in your mind, send the om outward to your friends in the circle, hear and feel their oms coming back to you, support the continuous sound when you take a breath, listen to the ups and downs, hear every voice, a little bit different but vibrating together to make a larger om that could just go on forever.

Let this be your last breath, aware of the vibration oming inside and outside of you. Let it go when you run out of breath (wait until it's quiet), and now take the power of that om with you for the rest of the day so you are able able to notice it anytime, anyplace.

———————— *

Discuss how the om could have gone on longer, how it was more powerful as a group than as individuals. Did people notice the sounds changing over time? Where in their bodies could people feel the sound and vibration? Can anyone still hear it in their mind or feel it vibrating in their body?

* *Practice 4.8: Integrating Mindfulness into Arts and Crafts*

There are a number of different ways to incorporate art and mindfulness practice. Many arts and crafts activities can be done in mindfulness. I worked briefly as a carpenter and, as the new guy, I was always assigned sanding, which I found to be incredibly boring. Eventually I began to move my body and hands together mindfully, truly feeling the surface beneath the wood as it changed; the work got a lot more interesting and a lot more enjoyable. Making prayer or wish flags is a fun activity that borrows from Himalayan tradition, and is an excellent way to say goodbye to a class or group. Each member writes a wish for themselves and everyone in the group and you string up all the flags. Asian or European calligraphy traditions, arts like *sumi-e*, origami, making mandalas, and even more familiar crafts like sculpture, painting, drawing, and flower arranging can be done mindfully, engaging several senses. I also keep some photocopies of mandala and fractal coloring books in my desk, and allow children to color these during our meetings. The soothing and absorbing qualities occupy and still their minds, and soon they forget how much they are talking. Drawing teachers often recommend exercises like drawing the spaces around objects rather than the objects themselves, a thought-provoking way to shift our usual perspective on the world. Showing a picture or object like a bouquet of flowers, then removing it and asking children to draw it from memory can be interesting. Singing, dancing, and chanting are other traditional forms of meditation that children can get involved in. Cooking is a fun opportunity to practice mindful awareness and so is mindful eating, especially when the vegetables come from your own garden, fertilized with your own compost. Painting and drawing can be done on homemade paper made from your own recycled materials. Craft books are a great place to look for inspiration and simply integrate mindfulness into the process.

Snow globes make tangible demonstrations of metaphors for settling the mind. Many craft stores sell snow globes into which you can place a picture of something or someone special. Even if you cannot find them, a few empty jars and some different colored glitter to represent thoughts, feelings, and sensations floating about in our consciousness make a perfectly good substitute. Some gold glitter can represent feelings, or other colors can represent thoughts or sensations, or different feelings. Children can mindfully choose to decorate and fill their snow globes with special items, and then gaze at them to help soothe and settle themselves as they watch the glitter settle.

* *Practice 4.9: Snow Globes*

Explain that our minds behave a lot like snow globes. As soon as we pick them up to examine them, we start noticing all these different things going on. Thoughts are swirling around like the white snow, feelings are swirling around like the silver snow, and they all look jumbled up and we don't know which is which or what they all mean. So we have to allow them to settle. The first thing to do is still the body, so we can still our mind. Set the snow globes down. Now, we can watch things settle. Just watch for a moment as things settle down. It may not take long in the snow globe the way it does in your mind, but you also can't make either settle without being still yourself. But just take time to let your mind settle. Now, shake your snow globe, follow just one of the pieces of glitter or snow as it travels. Be aware of your breath as you watch the storm in the globe simply calming itself. If you lose track of one piece of glitter, simply find another to watch swirl until it settles. As you watch, let your mind settle itself. When your snow globe settles, check in with your mind. Is it more settled than before? Try lifting and swirling the globe again.

* *Practice 4.10: The Magic Pendulum*

This exercise is a good way to calm down a child or a group and prepare them to focus, perhaps after a transition or before a test. The concept is quite simple.

Make a small pendulum, perhaps out of a necklace or a thin piece of string or fishing line, with a crystal, rock, or an I Ching coin tied to one end. Have the child hold the end of the string between the thumb and forefinger of one hand. With the same elbow resting on a table at about forty-five degrees, have them hold the pendulum just over a dot on a piece of paper. Have them breathe gently as they watch the compass still itself.

Try this script, or adapt it to fit the situation: Now, holding your hand and body perfectly still, and using only your mind, imagine the pendulum is beginning to swing gently from left to right. You don't need to move your hand at all, just use your mind and watch as the pendulum slowly starts to move...a little bit at first, then the motion becomes larger and larger. Once your mind has gotten your pendulum swinging left to right, see if your mind can move it so it is swinging front and back. Notice the pendulum start to change, slowly at first, until it begins moving in a forward and backward motion. Push with your mind as your fingers and arm remain perfectly still. Now watch the pendulum move up and down. Can you make it move in circles using only your mind? Try it, focus your mental energy on the pendulum once more, the up and down motion becomes an oval, widening outward, gradually it begins to move in a circle. Now see if you can make the circle smaller and smaller again. Now make tiny circles. And now stop the pendulum from moving with just your mind. Set your arm down and relax. As you come back, take with you the incredible power of your own mind, take with you, too, this feeling of relaxation and strength. You can return to it for the rest of the day.

Process the exercise with the children, how it felt and what might have surprised them. Can they use the power of their mind to do other things? This exercise quiets the mind for transition to doing work or talking about something that may require the concentration of a settled mind.

✻ *Practice 4.11: Zen Counting*

This is an old and fun summer camp activity that can build concentration and social awareness, reading nonverbal social cues and handling frustration. It also builds a sense of connectedness, since everyone loses or wins together. It can be a good way to start off a mindfulness group session, as games get people interacting and involved immediately.

A group of people stand in a circle, usually with eyes closed, and begin counting. Anyone can start, saying the number one but the same person can't then say two. Someone else has to say the next number, but if two people say it at the same time, start the count over. Try to get to twenty, or even ten, and discuss the frustrations and possible strategies that people could use without talking.

———————— ✻

This next exercise helps children not feel so alone when they're in a frightening or new situation, and can help all kinds of young people get in touch with their heritage with pride and gratitude. Have your children assume a comfortable sitting posture.

✻ *Practice 4.12: Greeting Visitors*[21]

If the tree is to flower, it must know its roots.
—West African proverb

Show your child or children pictures of a place their ancestors were from. If this is a school setting, each child could bring in a picture from home. It can be a photograph or something found in a magazine or online. Use this script or adapt it for your needs: For now, just focus on the breath, letting your belly go up and down as the air flows in and out. And now, imagine yourself in your ancestral homeland, perhaps a desert, a forest, a grassy plain, perhaps in the mountains, or by the ocean. Imagine yourself walking, taking in the sights, sounds, and smells.

You approach a river or stream and gently sit down on the bank. Sit yourself down comfortably. Feel the fresh air on your cheek, breathe in the air that your ancestors breathed. On your next breath, breathe deeply. Breathe out and everything becomes twice as colorful, the sounds twice as sharp. As you sit and breathe in your ancestral home, notice in the distance a figure walking toward you.

It is the spirit of your ancestors, here in human form, dressed in the traditional clothing of your ancestral people. This person looks a lot like you, but is grown and powerful, confident and strong. He or she smiles, and you smile back as the ancestor takes a seat beside you, and you two simply sit together.

While you sit, the visitor might tell you about his or her life, and even tell you about your own life as well. As you sit, you may notice your own thoughts. Watch these thoughts approaching, perhaps floating on the stream, perhaps coming by land. Greet each thought with the same openness and smile that you greeted your ancestor. Perhaps these thoughts are scary or unpleasant, notice this, but remember that your ancestors can and will protect you. A frightening thought might approach, but you know that the ancestor can defend you if you need help. Together you can smile and greet the thought, perhaps the thought sits and stays with you a while, caught in the river or sitting on the opposite bank for a while, but the thought always moves on. Or perhaps happy thoughts come by for a visit, you may want to invite them to stay, but they too cannot stay forever, eventually they walk or drift away, maybe to return, maybe not. You can simply greet each thought and then say farewell.

After a few minutes of greeting your thoughts, your ancestor tells you it's time to return to the room where you are. He or she reminds you that they are always with you, always here inside to answer your questions, to say hello and goodbye to anything that comes up. You can safely stand up for yourself with your ancestor there to protect you. Wiggle your toes and fingers, begin to stretch your arms and legs out and return to the room. Allow your eyes to gently open.

*

Following the exercise, you may want to ask the children to draw or write about their ancestor. Perhaps they want to share with the group, or they might prefer to keep it to themselves. You may suggest they keep a picture in their pocket for hard times.

The Six Senses or Nature Meditation

This next few meditations hone sensory awareness and insight into the interconnections of perceptions, thoughts, and feelings. Beginning with meditations that focus on the five senses is a concrete and accessible way to introduce children to mindfulness. To these five senses, the first exercise below adds a sixth sense: thoughts or perception.

This first exercise has been adapted for children with attention difficulties, as it shifts attention to different places quickly and is thoroughly guided. The purpose is to bring awareness to different sensations, and to our reactions to different sensations. Typically, we can think of these sensations as having three tones: pleasant, unpleasant, and neutral. Note how we respond differently in thought, emotion, and action to each one. It is amazing how often we desire change or want to keep grasping at what feels good.

This is a long exercise to do all at once, so depending on the child's age and attention span, it can be abbreviated or done in parts over time, using one sense for each time. Other variations are possible; I've done this as a "nature meditation" outside on a retreat in the Himalayas—gradually shifting awareness through the senses and tuning into one and then the next.

✻ *Practice 4.13: The Six Senses*

Have your children name the five traditional senses: smell, taste, touch, hearing, and sight. Then introduce them to a possible sixth sense: perception or thought. Ask them if they can categorize most of their reactions to these senses as pleasant, unpleasant, or neutral. Give some examples, such as the taste of ice cream as pleasant, the sound of someone screaming as unpleasant, the feel of a cotton shirt as neutral, and help your child or children think of some until you are sure they are clear on the idea. For this exercise you may want to draw a picture of a house with six windows; these are the windows of perception that allow us to perceive the outer world with those senses that we just named. Then, for each sense, follow the exercise below.

Part 1: Sight

Take a few moments to point out things in the children's line of sight, growing more detailed. At first glance, there might seem like there are only a few, say, red things in this room. Have your child guess how many and then look closer. Point out ones she or he may have missed. Now quietly count all the red things to yourself and have your child or children count all that they can find. With older children, you can go through more different colors of the rainbow.

Part 2: Hearing

Go outside or open the window if you are inside. Ask children to listen while "turning down" their other senses. Be quiet for a moment, and listen to the sounds of silence. After a few minutes of total silence, have the children quietly get out a piece of paper and write down the sounds they hear, everything. After a few minutes ask them to count how many sounds they heard. Have each child share one that hasn't been mentioned and have everyone go around once before anyone goes twice.

Part 3: Touch

Have your children close their eyes and try to sit still. First have them notice places on their bodies that are making contact or touching something. Starting with the feet, notice how they feel in their socks, perhaps tight or loose in their shoes, and gently resting upon the ground. Now have them notice their legs, where the skin makes contact with their pants, how does that feel? Does it tickle, feel scratchy, warm or cold, does it feel heavy? Do the sensations change? Now notice their bellies, perhaps they can feel them moving in and out, tightening against their shirts and pants. Again, is the feeling positive, negative, or neutral? How do their seats feel on the chairs under them? Comfy, not comfy? What are their hands making contact with? Is it something smooth or rough, pleasant or unpleasant? You can continue with this script, or adapt it for your situation: How does the air feel on your face and head? Notice where your lips touch…where your eyelids meet, where your nose and mouth touch the air…. Notice the cool air when you breathe in, the warm air as you breathe out. And now become aware of sensations inside your body, your tummy, your heartbeat. Thank your body for taking care of you. And now gently bring your awareness back from the feeling window and into the room.

Parts 4 and 5: Smell and Taste

Feel free to use this script or adapt it for your style and group:

Close your eyes and take a few moments to settle back with your breath. Notice the breath in your belly, and in your mouth and nose. What is the breath bringing you? First bring your awareness to your nose, noticing the cool air where it hits your nostrils. What are your breath and nose bringing you, telling you? Open your awareness to any smells that your nose-window may be bringing you. The odors in the room, the fresh air or not so fresh air… (name a few odors if present: food, the carpet, the plants). How do you experience them? Pleasant? Unpleasant? Neutral? Do any of them remind you of anyone or anyplace you've been before? Do you feel like you want them to be stronger or do you want to move away from them? Maybe they make you want to wrinkle your nose? What is your mind telling you to do?

Now bring your awareness to your mouth, and the air moving in and out of your mouth. Notice any tastes you might experience in your mouth. Maybe it's the taste of the air, maybe it's something you ate or drank earlier. This one is particularly hard, but see if you can just notice one thing, maybe on your tongue or in your cheeks. Maybe it's the lip balm on your lips. What does it feel like, and what does your mind do when it becomes aware?

Part 6: Thought

Use the following script or adapt it to fit the situation: Relax your eyes. Just for now, focus on your breathing. Keep your mind steady on where you most notice the breath coming and going in your body. Remain aware of sounds, of smells and tastes, the sensation of sitting…and when you are ready, imagine sitting next to a stream. When you watch the stream flowing by, notice what is flowing in the stream. Perhaps a leaf floats by, carried gently by the water. You can see it appear upstream, get closer as it flows past you, and then float downstream and out of sight once more. Each of your thoughts is like the leaf. Instead of following a thought that takes you away from the stream, just notice it. Notice the thought coming and then just return your attention to the stream, letting that thought go without traveling with it. When thoughts arise, set them on the leaf, and just let them float away, and then bring your thoughts back to the stream. You don't need to get on the leaf with the thought and follow its story—acknowledge it, and carefully place it on the leaf and let it float away. Sit for another moment noticing each thought as it comes. If a feeling arises, like a desire to itch or squirm, try to just set that on the leaf, notice if it feels positive, negative, or neutral, and let it flow away. If you forget and get on the leaf on its journey, just swim back to shore and start over again. Don't worry about how many times you want to go with the thought, you can always let go and swim back to shore. The current will always be strong and try to pull us along. If it's important, the thought will come back.

Now let's thank our six sense organs: the eyes for working hard to help us see, our ears always open to sounds around us, our nose to help us smell the flowers or tell us when food will be healthy, safe, and delicious, our taste buds to help us enjoy our food. Thank you to our bodies for taking care of us, letting us feel the earth. Thank you for the things and the people around us. And finally we thank our mind for our thoughts, which are, after all, only thoughts.

———————— *

This whole exercise in all parts can be done in nature turning up and turning down various senses, and so it works wonderfully on a family camping trip, a school field trip, or just a day at the park. If it's an inside day, it can also be combined with art activities that have kids writing or drawing pictures of what their senses noticed.

* *Practice 4.14 Everyday Mindfulness, Everyday Games*

One of my favorite ways to incorporate mindfulness into daily life with kids is by integrating it into existing games. I see a ten-year-old child named Jeffrey each week in my office. He has autism and an IQ so low that it wasn't measured. He struggles enormously with language and learning, as well as simply controlling his behaviors and impulses. Jeffrey is charming with an infectious smile and laugh, and although clumsy most of the time, can do the most incredible dance moves when we listen to music.

It is helpful to remind Jeffrey what he can do, rather than what he can't. Typically when we meet, we do some talking and check in about the past week and then I let him pick out a board game. Before each roll of the dice, however, we both take two mindful breaths, and then release the dice on the exhale. I'm convinced it leads to better rolls, and so is Jeffrey. He even suggested breathing in the feeling of getting a good roll and breathing out the bad feelings of getting a roll we didn't want. We also try to take one full breath before speaking, and focus on finishing our breath so that we truly listen and don't end up interrupting each other. With other children, in more strategic games (backgammon, checkers, chess, cards), we breathe fully and then try to see all of the options on the board before making a move. I know my backgammon skills have been improving, and I see fewer impulsive moves in many of the children I work with who stop and think before they act in games and in the rest of their lives. And they are always happy to remind me when I forget my deep breaths.

Just as we adults strive to bring a mindful awareness of the present in everything we do, children can aim for the same goal with our help. Assigning homework like getting in touch with the breath, or just stopping to notice one's thoughts at certain moments, will help children take mindfulness with them throughout the day. The breath, of course, is always with us. Many great teachers offer lists of good times to check in with the breath, such as at the first step of a stairwell, each time we touch a doorknob or lift a pencil, while tying shoes, waiting for video games to load, before looking at our buzzing telephone or certain sounds that we hear throughout the day. Classroom transitions are natural opportunities for walking meditation, and mindful activities can help children "shift gears" or settle into a new activity. Simple three-minute mindfulness activities like "The Breathing Space" and checking in with body, breath, and mind for just three breaths can be done at points throughout the day.[22] Mealtime is another opportunity; even just a mindful first bite or two is a valuable lesson and reminder.

Teachers can ask children to wait a mindful breath or two before or while raising their hand, taking a test, or doing a class presentation. Coaches can encourage children to take breaths before any games, teaching that the breath brings body and mind together and brings the mind back to the body. Impulsive children may do well to practice mindfulness during other children's turns at school or in games, when suppressing impulses can get difficult. And as children finish a project, I encourage them to think of something they are grateful for as they finish up their meditation, and to thank each other for support rather than displaying only pride in their accomplishment.

The meditations included here are only a few among dozens, if not hundreds, that will work with children. As you begin to practice with the children in your life, you will likely think of many more and be able to adapt many more. Mindfulness is referred to as a practice because, like anything else, it strengthens as we work on it. Children practice new skills all the time. With so many different ways to practice, children can choose what meditations work best for their unique learning style—play, the body, the senses, guided or self-led. Finding a meditation that fits means the child is more likely to stick with it and practice and strengthen his awareness. Gradually, as you and your children become more and more mindfully aware, it will become clear that this mindful awareness can be brought to anything. In fact, it will become a challenge to see where you cannot use it. The hardest part is remembering to get in touch with it and stay in touch with the present. After all, as Thich Nhat Hanh says, "the opposite of mindfulness is not mindlessness, but forgetfulness."

* 4.15 *One Hundred Things for Kids to Do Mindfully*

1. Breathe in. 2. Take a walk. 3. Stretch your arms. 4. Eat your favorite meal. 5. Smell the flowers. 6. Shoot some hoops. 7. Hug a friend. 8. Hug a tree. 9. Visit an animal shelter. 10. Work on a puzzle. 11. Write a poem. 12. Take a bath. 13. Listen to a friend. 14. Balance an egg on its end. 15. Listen to music. 16. Speak to a friend. 17. Make a list of your favorite things. 18. Draw or paint. 19. Sip some tea. 20. Listen to a friend's heartbeat. 21. Water your plants. 22. Play an instrument. 23. Hum or ommmm. 24. Try a yoga pose. 25. Dance. 26. Tell someone you appreciate her. 27. Work on a scrapbook. 28. Cook a meal. 29. Build a model. 30. Brush your teeth. 31. Sing! 32. Put on a good smelling lotion. 33. Look at your baby pictures, and your parents' baby pictures. 34. Make a list of people you are happy to have in your life. 35. Tense and release your muscles. 36. Feel the sunshine and breeze on your skin. 37. Wash your face. 38 Tie your laces. 39. Roll the dice in a game. 40. Plant a garden. 41. Wrap a present. 42. Build a sandcastle. 43. Doodle. 44. Practice calligraphy. 45. Brush your hair. 46. Peel and eat an orange. 47. Brush a friend's hair. 48. Finger paint. 49. Cook a meal and eat it. 50. Balance pennies on your shoes. 51. Use your non-dominant hand to write, draw, or brush your teeth. 52. Swing on a swing. 53. Slide down a slide. 54. Juggle. 55. Make a sandwich. 56. Watch the sunset. 57. Look for shooting stars. 58. Watch the clouds. 59. Build a fort with snow or pillows. 60. Play with your pets. 61. Paint your fingernails 62. Ski or snowboard. 63. Clean your room. 64. Walk with something balanced on your head or shoes. 65. Water your plants. 66. Watch the ripples on a pond. 66. Listen to the wind in the trees. 67. Lie in the grass. 68. Organize your photographs. 69. Teach mindfulness to a friend. 70. Smell different jars of spices. 71. Make a collage. 72. Give a back rub. 73. Do community service. 74. Go swimming. 75. Make and drink hot chocolate or lemonade. 76. Repair something broken. 77. Count your blessings. 78. Fly a kite. 79. Be kind to a stranger. 80. Make a card. 81. Shake a snow globe and watch the snow settle. 82. Smell perfume or candles. 83. Look through an art book or visit an art museum.

84. Explore your neighborhood. 85. Eat finger foods with a knife and fork. 86. Roller skate or skateboard. 87. Tune your instrument. 88. Shine your shoes. 89. Pat your head while rubbing your belly. 90. Make origami. 91. Sit by a stream. 92. Watch a sunset. 93. Find the constellations. 94. Rake leaves. 95. Listen to the sounds of nature. 96. Write a thank you note to a friend for being a good friend. 97. Write one to yourself. 98. Recite a poem. 99. Climb a tree. 100. Breathe out.

5

Practices for Mental Clarity and Creativity

Tell me, and I will listen. Show me, and I will understand.
Involve me, and I will learn.
—Lakota Proverb

Education is the soul of a society as it is passed from
one generation to the next.
—G. K. Chesterton

These days we may have books and computers to help us analyze and keep track of information, but meditative exercises have long been a key to learning and thinking creatively inside and outside of the classroom. Carefully honed meditative practices helped prepare the brains of Hindu and Muslim scholars to memorize the thousands of pages of scripture to pass on knowledge, long before most people could read or write. It seems impossible now to imagine systematically memorizing thousands of verses of scripture, but the reality is that one purpose of meditation was to train the brain so that these sorts of tasks were possible. Young people's brains today are not inherently different: they still have the same genetic makeup, and their minds have just been trained differently due to different cultural priorities in our contemporary society.

Contemplative practices led directly to the creativity and flexibility of thinking that allowed the North African Muslims to develop algebra. Remember that it was when Archimedes was taking a break in the bathtub, not while working at his desk, that he had his famous "Eureka!" moment. And it may only be a legend, but it is still revealing that Sir Isaac Newton was resting under a tree when a falling apple led to his insight about gravity. Quiet contemplation creates the conditions for new ideas and insights to arise. Monasteries East and West have always combined spiritual practice and quiet reflection with learning and creative innovation.

Meditation teacher Deborah Rozman describes the ways Eastern educators have used sense-awareness and other meditations to help students perceive and process information more effectively. She points out that in early childhood we listen and respond naturally and from the heart. We are actively curious and learn through all of our senses. Think of the small child whose favorite question is simply, why? and consider how that curiosity and openness gradually fades over time. We must begin to ask ourselves what we as parents and educators do that dampens this natural curiosity and openness, and try not to extinguish it.

As we get older, formal education and other aspects of our culture train us to discriminate in what we take in. This change brings many benefits in efficiency with learning but comes with many drawbacks. We learn to automatically and unconsciously dismiss certain valuable and creative ideas based on how school and culture have trained us to think.[23] But what is lost can be regained through mindfulness practice. A child can become more aware and interested in every thought—including what it is that they are missing—and empowered to choose to experiment rather than dismiss thoughts without conscious consideration. This is the very essence of creativity, or to use the cliché, thinking outside the box.

The best educators, from Plato to your favorite college professor, teach students how to teach themselves. They know that stoking creativity and curiosity are essential in training students to ask the right questions in order to get at the answers they seek. Whether we work in a classroom or not, we *will be* teachers if we spend time with children. Children are always students, always learning, whether explicitly or from our example. It is our responsibility to plant the seeds of curiosity and teach children how to water these seeds. As they begin to learn, we step back and allow them to harvest what we have given them.

Points of Contact Meditation

This exercise helps clear the mind and bring a sense of groundedness, and can be done for ten seconds or ten minutes. The start or end of a class period or the school day is a natural time to help children settle into their next activity by getting in touch with their bodies and then reconnecting with their minds and focusing.

Anchoring our focus on the entire body at once is a tall order, which is why it can be helpful to focus on certain points in the body where the breath is felt, move awareness through the body as in a body scan, or bring awareness to sensations in certain places. An easy place to find and to focus on is on our bodies' points of contact. These include where our bodies rest on the ground or cushion, usually our buttocks and legs, places where our body makes contact with itself, as with our hands, eyelids, lips, and legs, or where our skin makes contact with the air and clothes. At the Insight Meditation Society's Teen retreat, they suggest using the body, breath, or sounds as an anchor. The teen yogis usually focus on the hands, which they rest in each other or on the top of the legs.

* *Practice 5.1: Points of Contact*

Bring awareness to one particular part of your body and what it is touching. Allow this one point to be an anchor of awareness and focus on it as you breathe in and out. Notice what sensations you feel and the ways they change over time. The sensations may include awareness of weight, pressure, temperature, moisture, pulse and circulation, comfort or discomfort, and any other factors that make up the sensory experience of our hands or other part of the body.

A variation or second part to add is to make the point of contact a balancing challenge. Try balancing something on your head, or balancing coins on the tips of your shoes.

*

Academic Anxiety

One way that meditation can boost academic performance is by mitigating the effects of stress. Stress has a major impact on the performance of students as well as parents, teachers, or any professional. In some corners of our culture, we think of stress as good—it motivates us—or as a badge of honor that means you are a hard worker. The reality is somewhat more complex, and the relationship between stress, motivation, and performance is only true up to a certain point. Scientists describe the Yerkes-Dodson Curve, a mathematical graph that shows diminishing returns in cognitive performance after a certain level of arousal or anxiety. This is particularly true with efficiency, attention, problem solving, and memory.

Meditation can balance the ideal level of motivating stress with the openness that accompanies an optimal degree of calm. This balance explains studies that have found better performance in students who meditate or use other relaxation strategies. Relaxation allows those spontaneous moments of insight to arise, as with Archimedes in his bathtub and countless other "geniuses" who knew the value of contemplative relaxation. I talk often in meditation groups I've led about how stress is about being everywhere *but* the here and now—the mind is in the future, worrying about a test or a Friday night date that has not happened yet, or in the past, regretting what was written on yesterday's essay.

Mindfulness brings us into direct contact with the here and now, and with practice gives students a choice about whether to, as one of my students put it, "worry about being worried about being stressed for the exam" or just make an effective study plan for that big test next week and to focus on the next step in front of them. The research has found academic improvement in terms of executive functioning, attendance, and improved social skills after a five-week mindfulness curriculum. Research by Dr. Herbert Benson even discovered that teachers who meditate or use relaxation techniques have higher performing students.

The Shaolin monks of China and Mongolia once developed a special practice to relax into learning. They lived in the mountains, far from other people, and every year watched the seasons change and looked forward to springtime in the high plateau. The protective snow would melt, revealing the green plains and bringing fresh food and flowers. The wet plains would then dry up and evaporate into the clouds above, returning to nature only to return again the following winter. This exercise is adapted from their story.

✻ *Practice 5.2: Ice, Water, Vapor*[24]

Use this script with your child or adapt it as needed:

First, sit or lie down comfortably. Focus on your breath gradually letting thoughts slip away, feeling comfortable yet strong. Be aware of the places your body is making contact with the chair or ground around you, your feet, arms, and seat. Gently close your eyes when you feel ready. Return your awareness to the breath, not forcing it, just letting your body breathe for you. Notice that you don't even have to breathe, your body takes care of you and all you have to do is watch. As you breathe, follow your breath down into your toes and feet. Notice the tension in your feet, feeling frozen solid and heavy like a block of ice in the mountains. As you breathe in sunshine, feel your feet gradually melting into a puddle, each breath bringing warmth and relaxation until the frozen blocks that are your feet have turned into puddles. Now with each breath, let the puddles dry into steam, evaporating into clouds.... With the next breath, feel the cloud that was once your feet drifting away in the breeze, rejoining with nature.

Now notice your lower legs, frozen, heavy, and now the breath begins to melt the ice that is your legs, turning to snow, and feel the relief as it melts away like a snowman in the sun. The puddle of water evaporates into steam and now floats away into the air. Now feel your heavy thighs and knees, weighed down with tension so tight it could snap like ice. Now let your breath melt the ice before it breaks, relaxing, dripping down into a pool of water, gradually becoming vapor in the air. And with the next breath it is carried off, merging with the rest of the air.

Now feel your hips frozen like a glacier; with each breath they slowly melt and drip down into liquid, liquid turning to a cloud and drifting away on the summer breeze. Your lower back may feel frozen and heavy, the organs of your stomach chunks of ice set into a frozen snow bank, and now the healing breath breaks through the ice, melting, melting, turning to slush and dribbling into a puddle. The puddle dries up in the sun and floats away.

Bring your awareness now to the chest and upper back feeling heavy and numb, dripping into liquid, that liquid into steam and gradually joining with the air around you. Now let your frozen arms begin to melt from ice to water to air. Your neck and shoulders gradually let the tension and stiffness drain out with the breath flowing into liquid, evaporating into a light mist and now feel your frozen head, weighed down and heavy, beginning to melt with each breath. Feel it become slush, trickles of water now giving way to a puddle of cold liquid, the liquid warming and evaporating into a small cloud now where your head once lay. Letting go, the breath now carries the cloud into the air to rejoin the other parts of your body, drifting through the air completely relaxed and letting the wind carry your body away, leaving just your breath and your thoughts. Now let go of the thoughts leaving just the breath, just follow the breath now. (Pause for a few moments or for a few minutes.)

And now allow the clouds to slowly re-form into the shape of your body, becoming solid now, but restored without any of the tension of before, gradually returning to yourself with a freshness that you didn't have before, a fresh awareness and fresh body that you can carry with you the rest of the day. Wiggle your fingers and toes and stretch your body to make certain it is solid. Gradually turn on your side and take the relaxation with you, and now sit up.

Attention and Academic Performance

Our children are coming of age in a culture that constantly demands they fragment their attention rather than train their ability to concentrate on a task. Mindfulness practice trains the mind to be aware of the different trains of thought without becoming distracted or derailed by them.

In his book *The Mindful Brain*, Daniel Siegel writes about studies that show that mindfulness training has a role in strengthening attention and executive functioning through changing neural pathways. Other researchers found similar results, as well as improved attention span in adults and teens with and without ADHD.[25] Brain-scan studies have also found attention regions activated and strengthened in meditators.[26] Even brief mindfulness exercises before an attention test seemed to improve performance, suggesting that a brief mindfulness exercise could greatly improve test performance or concentration for studying.[27] More promising research continues to emerge almost daily, even as this book goes to publication.

✻ *Practice 5.3: Sound Awareness*

With older children and adolescents, I like to make this exercise something of a game, though some young people can certainly become more competitive than others, so beware. Begin the lesson by writing the word "silent" on the board. Ask your students to rearrange the letters to form a new word. (Have you guessed it yet yourself?) It spells "listen." Lead a brief discussion about the importance of listening and the role that silence can play in helping us to listen to the world, to ourselves, and to strengthen our attention, then hand out some paper and pencils.

✻

The Sound Sense

Now we will open the window of sound and listening. Do you think there will still be noise when we are completely quiet? Silence is silence, right? Well, we'll find out. We will be quiet for a moment, and listen to the sounds of silence. If your mind starts to wander, just gently notice where it goes and bring your attention back to your ears. Quietly get out a piece of paper and write down the sounds you hear, everything. When I say go, start listening carefully and quietly. (Wait about a minute, writing down what you hear as well.) How many people heard nothing in the silence? How many people heard one thing, raise your hand? Two things? Three or more? Okay, let's hear them. (Go around the room asking for sounds, perhaps starting with those children who you expect may have more difficulty.) So, now we have way more sounds than we ever thought were there. Let's all listen together for another moment and see what else we can hear. (Listen for another minute or so, then discuss the exercise and its implications about noticing things that we weren't aware of before bringing our attention to them.)

With an older or more experienced group, I'll often add a few variations. One variation is asking people in the second part to not just note what they hear, but what association, thought, or feeling (if any) comes up right afterward, and then returning to the listening. One student commented with wonder at how many little joys and sorrows and frustrations she must be having all day that never enter her conscious awareness, just based on sounds. This led to a great discussion. Another variation is to ask students to listen to the spaces between sounds, to try to find the true silence. Still another variation is to use these two sound awareness exercises as a springboard for spending a few minutes listening to the "mind sense" and just noting what thoughts arise.

This sound listening is an interesting assignment that I often practice with both kids and adults, who have found it helpful in different ways. One friend who practiced with her anxious daughter described the relief her daughter expressed after practicing this at a slumber party. Her daughter focused on the sounds of laughter around her and realized she didn't need to be nervous; she could just be aware of how much fun everyone was having and know it was okay.

But other people may have different responses. I worked with a kid named Andy in a very chaotic special education school who had a terribly difficult time with his emotions and a history of trauma and hallucinations. Andy and I practiced the exercise together in the therapy room, while in the hallway we could hear children and adults literally screaming. I asked him what he noticed. "Screaming. I'm scared." I agreed, we were in a very scary school that often felt unsafe. Andy confessed that when there was so much screaming the voices in his head sometimes got louder and he couldn't tell what was real. He wanted to keep listening though, so we gave it another minute. I would gently remind him every few seconds to notice the sound and the thoughts he had, but then go back to the sound and away from the thoughts. We checked in again after the minute was up. "It's scary in this school," he said again. "And sometimes I hear kids screaming, and I think that could be me, and I get upset in class and can't control my behaviors anymore. But right now I hear it and I feel scared, but I also know I'm okay and safe in here with you." I tell this story because a lot of these exercises can sometimes be more overwhelming before they become helpful, and it is so important to keep in mind who you are working with and what environment you are working in.

Creativity, Awareness, and Acceptance

Knowledge is limited, but imagination encircles the world.
—Albert Einstein

Another important psychological function of mindfulness and meditation is in creating cognitive flexibility and awareness, key aspects of creativity.[28] Creativity is a vital quality not just in artistic endeavors but in school and life. Think of the creativity demanded in leadership, problem-solving on micro and macro levels, as well as effective self-expression.

This exercise, adapted from a Chinese folktale, teaches the value and wisdom of acceptance of things as they are, as well as engages children's natural creativity. I tell one version here, but there are many more out there, including a beautiful illustrated version by Jon Muth in the book *Zen Tales* that would be better read aloud.

✻ *Practice 5.4: Sai and the Horse*

In ancient China lived an old farmer named Sai. He awoke one morning and looked in his stable, only to find that his horse had disappeared. He looked everywhere, but couldn't find it. His neighbors came by that afternoon to express their sadness at his apparent misfortune and bad luck. Sai took it in stride. "Bad luck, good luck who ever knows?" he asked them. A few days later his horse returned, this time with a mare. His neighbors congratulated him. "Sai," they exclaimed, "congratulations on your luck! You have two horses now!" "Bad luck, good luck, who ever knows..." he responded. A few weeks later, he awoke to the sound of his son crying outside. He ran out to find his son crying and holding his broken leg—he had just been thrown by the mare. His son lay in bed for weeks and the neighbors again came by and clicked their tongues. "What bad luck!" they exclaimed. "Bad luck, good luck, who ever knows?" said Sai. The next day the army came through town to take every young man to war, and the neighbors exclaimed again about the luck that Sai's son wasn't drafted for the war. So what do you think Sai said? "Bad luck, good luck, who ever knows?".

If you are using this story as an exercise with a group or reading it to your children, you can have the children each add another chapter to the story, with each child building on what happened in the chapter told by the student before. You can incorporate relevant themes from their lives, or ask them to do so. Record the stories on paper or through artwork.

Classroom or Group Management and Focus

A few moments of mindfulness each day can be a powerful reminder to children to refocus, prepare for transitions, and calm the body and mind. Rather than sharply disciplining children for a lack of focus, which is *reacting* to an existing behavior, mindfulness practice helps children *proactively* focus and prepare themselves. Get creative as you think about times and spaces in the busy week to integrate a few practices; a few minutes of mindful activities once a day or even a few breaths will likely pay off in the long run. A quick breathing exercise is just to practice diaphragmatic breathing and works fast to bring anxiety down and focus scattered energy.

Typically, we don't pay very much attention to the way we breathe, though with practice we start to change that. Most of the meditations in this book don't call for consciously changing the breath, though this exercise in breathing does ask for a deliberate shift. When we are anxious, which may be more often than we realize, we tend to breathe short, shallow breaths into the chest. We don't get the oxygen we need—thus lacking the energy we need for whatever is at hand—and we do not feel relaxed. When we breathe from our diaphragm, we are getting the oxygen that we need.

✳ *Practice 5.5: Belly Breathing*

The easiest way to move the breath into the diaphragm is to place one hand on the chest and one on the belly. This can be done either sitting or lying down. Breathe naturally, and notice which hand moves up and down. Simply try to gently move the breath further down with each breath until it is the belly that is moving up and down. Some people find it helpful to imagine a waterfall carrying the breath downward.

———————— ✳

A Classroom Explanation of Mindfulness and Meditation

Bring the class's attention to the chalkboard or whiteboard. Explain that each day you write on the board and then erase what you have written every few minutes or after each lesson. You can probably easily demonstrate this on your own board. By the end of the lesson, the board is clear from erasing, but there are bits of earlier lessons still showing through behind the most recent writing. Chalk or marker dust still clings to the board here and there. At the end of the day, or for some of us the end of the week, we get out the spray bottle and thoroughly clean the board to get rid of all those little bits and start fresh. Of course, we also have to remember to thoroughly clap out and clean our erasers every once in a while too. This is what meditation does; it's a cleaning of the board and our erasers to prepare us for what comes next, without the remnants of another day seeping through and making things hard to see. The mindfulness bell is our spray bottle. We might want to mindfully review the day's lessons as we clean, or we might want to simply erase, as in concentration meditation.

Other metaphors might include defragmenting your hard drive. Washing windows is another concrete metaphor that can also be demonstrated with a visual aid. Ask the children to look through a dusty piece of plastic or even a pair of goofy sunglasses, then clean the surface together and look through it again, reminding them of the value of cleaning and clearing their minds.

* *Practice 5.6: Following the Sound of the Bell*

A mindfulness bell is a very simple way to clear the mind. The best bells have an extended tone that lasts for a minute or longer. A simple souvenir bell or even a metal bowl will work, though the best are the iron bowls designed to hold an extended tone. In meditative traditions, we "invite" the bell to sound, rather than striking it. Hold the bell and take a few mindful breaths until you feel the bell has invited you to gently sound it.

Sitting quietly, ask the children to simply breathe and listen as you invite the bell. Ask them to quietly raise their hand when they can no longer hear the reverberations.

Invite the bell to sound, and discuss the sounds that people heard, the shape and tone of the sound, and the way it changed as it faded. Invite the bell again, and see if people notice more and different tones this time. You can use this as a way to introduce the bell to your class or family. Let your children know that every time they hear the bell sound, they should stop what they are doing and take three mindful breaths, focusing their attention on the sound of the bell until it fades, then return to their tasks. You might want to incorporate the bell at transitions or other points of the day. Before tests or presentations is a good time to practice. You can include children in your classroom by rotating who gets to invite the bell.

*

Building and Strengthening Emotional Intelligence

With the controversies of "the culture wars" in America, it can be hard to agree on how to teach values to our children. The diversity that makes our society strong also leads to disagreement not just on how to teach values, but on what values to teach. Still, most agree that we could be doing a better job. I believe that we can sidestep concerns about teaching right or wrong values by helping children increase their emotional intelligence, an idea popularized by Daniel Goleman. Below I have included a simple yet elegant concept from Marsha Linehan, who designed a straightforward model for making sense of our minds that was initially written for adults but is elegantly simple enough to be understood even by children. Her therapy model, dialectical behavior therapy, includes many elements of mindfulness. It empowers people to understand their emotions instead of being controlled by them. Her model explains states of mind as a Venn diagram—with reasonable mind and emotional mind overlapping in wise mind. Below is an outline of her lesson, which can be found in the book, *Skills Training Manual for Treating Borderline Personality Disorder*.

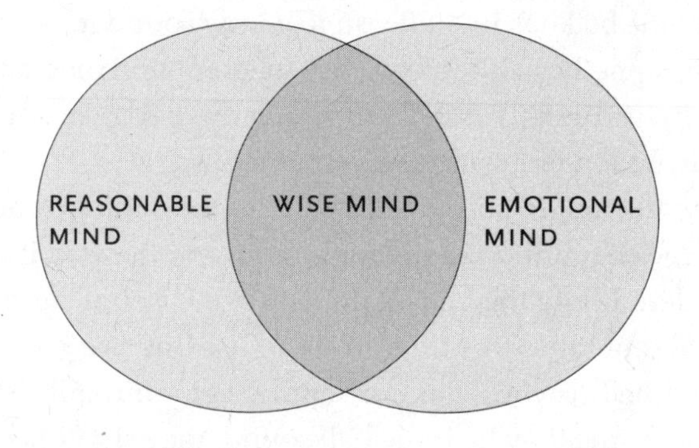

* *Practice 5.7 Wise Mind*[29]

Older children, adolescents, and teenagers often relate to these concepts. Draw the above diagram and then focus first on the definitions and uses of reasonable mind and emotional mind. Linehan explains the times and ways that our reasonable/rational mind is useful to us—in math class, when mapping out a trip, or solving certain kinds of problems that call for logic and cognition. There are also times when our emotional mind is effectively in control. Examples are making art or romantic literature and songs, dancing, and building relationships. But too much rational mind can also mean being coldly calculating, and too much emotional mind can include red-hot emotions that cloud our thinking and behavior. If you are doing this with a class, they can come up with their own examples. This can also lead to a discussion of what the pros and cons of these two states are and what emotional mind or rational mind feels like, using adjectives, colors, or metaphors in words or in drawings. Are these states sharp or soft, strong or weak, red or blue?

Wise mind is the ideal integration of these two states of mind. These are the times when we can listen to our emotions, listen to our logic, weigh them each, and be most likely to act in a skillful way. Help the group think of some examples of times they have felt in wise mind, and ways that they could access their wise mind as they think about difficult situations coming up. You may want to make a large poster, and write in words or examples, or cut out pictures for each section of the diagram and hang it in the classroom or community space.

What younger children may grasp with the simplicity of some of the earlier sensory exercises, older children may like in the analysis of the Wise Mind lesson. No matter how old your children are, mindfulness can be incorporated into lesson plans, large and small, for almost any subject. Ongoing classroom projects can include recording extended lists of what people hear during "silence" or a gratitude list that grows each day as people contribute one or two things they are grateful for to the list. Smaller mindfulness exercises like the bell can be simple reminders to focus and be in touch with the worlds inside and outside, leading to students who are happier and more aware of school and of life.

6

Practices for Physical Health

Our own physical body possesses a wisdom which we who inhabit the body lack.
—Henry Miller

TRADITIONAL MEDICINE from around the world has relied on meditative techniques to assist with the healing process for centuries; in fact, the words "meditation" and "medicine" even derive from the same Sanskrit root for inner measure. Recent science suggests that meditation and similar practices may be tapping into the body's own natural healing powers.[30] Meditation has been used not just to help heal the sick body, but also to strengthen healthy bodies, training athletes of today and warriors of the past. To suggest that meditation can cure serious diseases would be untrue, but meditation can be a powerful adjunct to the healing process, helping the immune system and certainly improving quality of life for those suffering with chronic illness, especially with symptoms like chronic pain and insomnia.

Herbert Benson, in *The Relaxation Response*, proposes a three-part model of healing. One part consists of modern medications, another includes physical treatments like surgery, and the third discusses "self-healing" activities like relaxation or meditative activities that trigger the body's natural healing mechanisms. We often think about the body's fight or flight mechanism for handling stress, in which our heart rate, breathing, and metabolism increase with an accompanying release of stress hormones. In recent years we have come to see that an opposite "relaxation response" also exists to heal ourselves. The modern world is filled with stresses like school, family, and relationships. The stress of applying to college is hardly life threatening, but the bodies we've inherited may react as if it is. We know that stress exacerbates both mental and physical illness, and meditation can play a strong role in reducing these complications. But meditation has been proven to do far more than just reduce stress.

Numerous studies have found mindfulness meditation helps boost the immune system, leading to more antibodies when exposed to influenza vaccine than control groups, or leading to faster rates of recovery from skin diseases like psoriasis and even lower frequency of colds, viruses, and headaches.[31] Other research shows lowered heart rate, blood pressure, metabolic rate, and breathing rate associated with meditation practice.[32] Though many of these are not childhood health problems, they offer hope that if begun early, meditation could offset some of the concerns about the future health of our children. Other promising studies link meditation and relaxation techniques to reductions in asthma, allergies, and even diabetes. Relaxation, body scans, and body awareness meditations are particularly effective in improving general physical health . The following meditation is a gentle relaxation exercise than can be done to calm down before bed or to soothe anxiety about the body, and can be practiced anywhere, even a frightening place like a hospital.

Children respond to this breathing meditation because it uses both physical and visual objects of concentration, as well as because it is fun. Using origami boats that the class makes as a mindful activity is a wonderful introduction into the exercise and leaves children with a physical reminder of mindfulness that they can take home with them or display in the classroom. The fact that this meditation requires lying down makes it an excellent choice for children who may be sick, bedridden, or partially immobilized.

✻ *Practice 6.1: Riding the Waves*

Invite the children to lie down on the floor, with their heads comfortably propped up with pillows so that they can watch their bellies. Have the children place a simple piece of paper, folded in half and opened up as a V, on their bellies in a way that it will not fall off.[33]

Sailors from all over the world and across history have understood the ocean as a powerful yet wise force. The ocean can be a frightening place. Waves can knock the largest boats off balance and sink them. But though we all can imagine the rise and fall of waves on the sea, we remember water always finds an even level in the end. Deep below the roughest seas lies a profound calm on the ocean's floor. Like the surface of the earth, our bodies are made mostly of water. For that reason, we too have the wisdom of water within each of us if we can find it. That calm can exist deep below a stormy surface, that calm can exist deep below even as rain and wind and lightning create dangerous waves.

Use this script and adapt as desired: Lie down comfortably where your eyes can watch your belly. Place your boat on your belly, allowing it to balance, and gently put your hands back on the ground facing upward, allowing them to gently relax and fall to the side if that is their natural state. Without changing your breathing, bring your attention to your breath, feeling the air flowing from your nose down through your throat and into your belly. Notice the way your belly and the ship on your belly rise with each breath. Just try to maintain your attention here, on the rise and fall of your belly. Notice the sensations of the breath, how it changes and adjusts without you even needing to think about it. Notice the way your body is held by the earth, like an ocean. The surface may go up and down, may speed up and slow down, but inside, the bottom of the ocean is calm, far away from the waves on the surface. Just remain aware of each breath. In and out. The sound is like the sound of the surf. When your attention wanders, just return to the breath, return to your boat rising and falling, always aware of the stillness underneath.

Up and down, rising and falling. Life's ups and downs don't need to take you off course or knock you off balance, you can even become comfortable in the ups and downs. Things will settle and we don't ever need to be knocked off balance. Return to the breath, the ups and downs of the breath calming you, centering you. The boat isn't in charge of the ups and downs, but remains steady with them. Focus on the sensation of breathing, notice the air in your nose and mouth. Feel the air lift your belly, just watch your belly and your boat for a few moments. Be aware of how it feels, aware of your mind. Continue for a few more moments of quiet breathing.

Set your boat at your side, and take with you the feeling of calm, remembering your breath as you turn onto your side, stretch, and gently sit up.

6.2 *Homesickness Meditation*

This exercise is often helpful for kids who become anxious when away from home—on school trips, at camp, the hospital, or even just sleepovers at friends' houses or anywhere they might feel homesick.

In my twenties, I spent a lot of time traveling in Latin America, India, Southeast Asia, and North Africa often on my own. Alone in a hostel or a strange town or train station, it was often frightening and overwhelming, hard to get my bearings to feel safe. With time, I became more able to "see" the parallels between my home and these seemingly exotic places where different languages were spoken and the cultural gap had seemed too wide to bridge. The bustling outdoor market was just the same thing as my local supermarket, the strange smells of foreign food were, well, just food. For kids spending the night away, it is helpful to look around and see what is the same, even if it looks different. This kitchen is different, but it's still a kitchen where the family hangs out to cook and eat like my family, even if it's a different color and different food. The soap and toothpaste in the bathroom smell funny, but they wash and clean my teeth just like in my home. The parents may look different, but they still love their kids. I have a clock in my room and so does my friend!

Making parallels, looking for similarities rather than differences can help the unfamiliar feel familiar, and show our interconnection. It is so helpful when meeting new people or encountering new situations to find out what we have in common; it makes us more connected, at ease, and less fearful. So encourage kids to take a few minutes to find what is familiar in strange situations.

*

Mindfulness and Food Consumption

Eating meditations are a wonderful and simple introduction to mindfulness for children and wonderfully engage all of our senses. They offer many lessons about our body, our mind, and our impulses. Mindful eating can be done at any meal, though maybe just try once a week to incorporate a short mindful eating practice with children. I do know a family with a school-phobic child who mindfully eats breakfast together in order to help the child stay calm before she has to go to school. Bringing mindfulness to many of the morning's routines can serve a similar purpose, from tooth-brushing to showering, to eating and packing the schoolbag. Meditation teachers for years have spoken of the benefits to mind and body when slowing down to eat, and research is showing that it does seem to help with gastrointestinal issues like irritable bowel syndrome, and even leads to the release of more digestive enzymes.[34] There have even been a few mindfulness-based eating programs that have been shown to reduce binge eating, a leading cause of obesity, as well as a variety of other eating disorders like bulimia and anorexia.[35]

It is easy to point fingers about the cause of the obesity crisis in our country but hard to pinpoint its roots exactly. However, one thing is clear, that we can individually take responsibility for what we put into our bodies, and we can help young people understand the importance of this as well. I recently worked with a young girl named Tamara who was very lonely and unhappy. She had long black braids and was always stylishly dressed with perfectly manicured fingernails. She used food as a comfort and would mindlessly eat chips, ice cream, and junk food after school when she had no friends to comfort her after a hard day at school. This was often followed by a hard afternoon at home where she lived alone with her angry and depressed mother after her father died.

Tamara and I together learned and practiced some basic mindful eating, and she was able to discover the joyous dimensions of food and eating, not just the numbing emotional effects. She proudly announced her discovery to me: "If I eat mindfully, I eat less and like the food more." Through her own process of mindful awareness, she had learned this on a much deeper level than if an adult had simply told her to slow down and eat less. Even just following the advice of our grandparents and chewing our food forty or fifty times before swallowing—watching this experience and being mindful of the urges that come with it—will slow us down and teach us so much about our own too-often-mindless relationship with food.

Finally, food also connects us to each other, to our ancestors and our culture of origin, and to our planet. Seeing where our food grows, especially by planting our own gardens is a true miracle, especially for children to witness. And taking a moment to consider where our food comes from, the people involved, brings us closer together with a greater awareness of our interbeing on this planet.

✻ *Practice 6.3: Five Contemplations on Eating*

The Five Contemplations that Thich Nhat Hanh recommends using at meal times are:

* This food is a gift of the earth, the sky, numerous living beings, and much hard work.
* May we eat with mindfulness and gratitude so as to be worthy to receive it.
* May we recognize and transform our unwholesome mental formations, especially our greed, and learn to eat with moderation.
* May we keep our compassion alive by eating in such a way that we reduce the suffering of living beings, preserve our planet, and reverse the process of global warming.
* We accept this food so that we may nurture our brotherhood and sisterhood, strengthen our Sangha (community), and nourish our ideal of serving all beings.

The classic eating exercise below is similar to the raisin exercise described in Chapter 4, though it goes through the whole process of eating the raisin or other item. In this case, I've used a grape with seeds, as it's nice to use a piece of fresh fruit.

✻ *Practice 6.4: Eating Meditation*

Hand out grapes to the group, and have them study the grapes for a few minutes, examining them in the light, playing with them in their fingers, bringing them up to their lips and watching themselves salivate. Then, gently, without biting into it, set the grape on your tongue, and notice any urges that come up. Notice what your tongue and mouth do or want to do as you taste the grape. Take a few moments now before you bite into the fruit, feeling its texture on your tongue and mouth, noticing the taste of its skin. When you are ready, bite into the grape, noticing the flavors and textures. As you continue to taste, try not to swallow yet. See if you can find the seed in the grape. What becomes of that tiny seed? What does it taste like? Keep tasting, noticing the sensations and thoughts that arise. How is your stomach feeling? And the rest of your body? When you are ready, go ahead and swallow the grape, noticing what you do and what your mouth does. After swallowing, take a moment and notice any leftover flavor remaining in your mouth, sensations in your stomach, and thoughts in your mind.

✻

Discuss the exercise with children afterward, inquiring about what was challenging, what people noticed or discovered, what people learned about the mind-body connection. Why does the first bite taste so good when we are eating, then after a time we stop noticing and just eat automatically, and by the end of the meal we forget how good that first bite was? You may want to suggest that they try this with their first bite of lunch that afternoon or dinner that evening, and check in again the following day.

Athletic Performance

Meditations have been and remain a part of physical health and athletics. World-class contestants, when they are interviewed, describe that when competing at such a high level, there is so little difference between the competitors' bodies that it becomes a mental game in which a well-trained mind can offer the edge. Body-based meditations like body scans or movement meditations help build that bodily awareness and kinetic intelligence while simultaneously sharpening awareness of one's surroundings. This allows a person to respond to the body's natural signals and care for her body, while anticipating what is coming next in the competition, "reading the field." And as a person cares for their body, so the body cares for that person.

The best athletes have been well-known to study other disciplines to more closely know their bodies. Boxers study dance, divers train in martial arts, basketball players practice breathing and visualization, and soccer players learn yoga to become more intimate with their greatest physical tool. Children may also respond better to focusing on movements rather than simply sitting or standing. Yoga, tai chi, qigong and other martial arts exercises are simple and fun entry points into greater bodily awareness. A simple mindful standing yoga exercise that enhances bodily awareness can be found in *The Mindful Way Through Depression* by Mark Williams.

Capoeira is an Afro-Brazilian martial art with a long history, originally created by African slaves hundreds of years ago. The slaves hid their powerful techniques from plantation owners by practicing them as a form of dance, explaining its grace. Through capoeira, it is thought that the Africans communicated, played, and practiced self-defense against their captors. The practice taught them respect for themselves, responsibility and empowerment for their family and friends, and cleverness of mind with the various ways they could adapt and disguise their power, giving them the key to their own freedom. After slavery ended, when the authorities realized the power of what they had thought was a game, they outlawed capoeira and it went underground. Eventually, the politicians realized the beauty of the art and soon recognized it as the national sport of Brazil. Today, capoeira is still practiced in Brazil, and all over the world competitions are held not to fight but to show skill. Spectators stand in a circle called a *roda*, cheering and listening to music that sets the pace of the movements. Capoeira academies train the mind and body to defend themselves. Masters impart values of respect (*respeito*), responsibility (*responsibilidade*), safety (*seguranca*), cleverness (*malicia*), and freedom (*liberdade*).

* *Practice 6.5: Capoeira Body Awareness*

The basic movement is called the *ginga*, which means simply rocking back and forth. Stand in a circle, or roda, far enough apart that you don't bump into one another, remembering the values of responsibility and safety. Standing with the feet shoulder width apart, step one foot back and forward again, then the other foot. Gently rocking this way, try to get into a rhythm and balance. As you move, think about the three points of a triangle that your feet are making. Feel your feet landing safely on the earth beneath you. Notice your body getting into a rhythm, that it naturally will balance you, even as you move. Trust your body. Notice sensations in the legs—can you feel the blood moving? Perhaps your heart beat is rising and your breathing is growing faster.

After a few minutes of practice, add your arm movements in. As the right foot steps back, the right arm and elbow should go up to chest level in a blocking manner. When the left foot goes back, the left arm moves up. At first they may feel stiff and awkward, but gradually you will begin to feel the rhythm. You are not competing, so remember to have respect for yourself and those around you. Feel the freedom in the movement. Notice the changes in your body, and the feelings of power and freedom that come to your mind. Stay on task: if your mind wanders, so will your rhythm, and then you won't be able to move as well. After a few minutes of practice, you may want to add in a drumbeat, allowing the drum to set the pace of the movement, letting it grow steadily faster. Follow the beat of the drum, but remain aware of your body to keep in time. Always stay aware of your space and those around you, so that everyone is safe and having fun.

———— *

For physical health and performance, the body requires a healthy and clear mind. For mental health and optimal cognitive functioning, the body must be a solid foundation, well-nourished and cared for, healthy and in good shape. With people of all ages, the evidence is mounting that physical health and mental health go hand in hand, as do physical and mental performance. Meditation and mindfulness can train each of these aspects of the whole person, bringing the person into wholeness from states of weakness, from suffering and confusion to states higher than we can imagine.

7

Practices for Mental and Emotional Well-being

Mind is a forerunner of all things. As we think and act, so our world becomes.
—THE DHAMMAPADA

IN RECENT YEARS, the surgeon general estimated that one in five American children and teens will suffer from some form of mental illness. Their suffering, in turn, profoundly impacts families, friends, schools, and our wider communities. Most of these are anxiety disorders, followed by behavior problems, then mood problems and others.[36] Clearly these are worrisome numbers, especially because this rate is rising against an overburdened mental health system. This sad state of affairs often leads to medications as a first line of treatment. By some estimates, upward of six million American children now take prescription medication daily. Confusion and controversy among experts about the proper diagnosis of children abounds, further complicating the situation.

To understand how mindfulness can help, it's useful to understand the causes and conditions under which mental health and emotional problems arise. Competing theories abound, but what is clear is that certain events and influences in our lives, combined with our genetic programming, can lead us into habitual thought patterns about ourselves and the world around us. These repeating "tapes" we play in our heads are often established in childhood and become deeply ingrained in our psyche and wired into our brain by the time we reach adulthood. They drive us to grasp after some things and avoid others, too often unaware of why we ever started reacting in these ways in the first place. Often these strategies relieve the pain, but at other times they lead us into more trouble. Over time, however, these patterns become physiologically hardwired.

Our neural pathways form into ruts that are not always helpful. Imagine a dirt road that ambles across a meadow. The road is worn down over the years by trucks repeatedly driving over the same tracks. We continue to drive on this path because it has been worn down, and it becomes more firmly established with each pass. This is exactly why we get stuck in old thoughts, feelings, and behaviors. Now imagine for a moment that a gentle rain comes and softens the whole field. With soft ground, creating a fresh and more direct path is that much easier. Mindfulness is like the rain that falls on the meadow, softening the ground to make blazing a new path easier. In time, we take the new path simply because it is there, and it becomes worn in deeper each time we drive down it.

Current psychological explanations mesh well with traditional spiritual explanations of how mindfulness operates. They suggest that psychological problems emerge out of "negative thought schemas," our habitual ruts. Mindfulness, unlike some other therapies, doesn't aim to change the thoughts. Rather, mindfulness practice seeks to change our relationship to the thoughts, while building cognitive flexibility, essentially creating space for other perspectives to enter our awareness. We are now empowered with a choice of various paths to take, no longer limited to the one we usually take. We come to realize that the old path is not the only option; it's just the one that we've grown accustomed to. We may also notice how scary it can be to try a new path until it becomes familiar.

Gradually, it becomes clear that anxious or depressed thoughts and feelings are mere events created by the brain and are by nature impermanent. We can't necessarily change the thoughts, but we don't need to believe them either. We can choose how we respond to these thoughts rather than instantly reacting to them. Gradually, thought patterns begin to change, and new thoughts emerge that are based on the reality around us rather than conditioned habits.

This is not to say that we should never believe our thoughts, it's just that we can learn to be aware of the contexts in which they arise. We cannot see in the fog or hear a bird's song over a loud garbage truck. Similarly, there are times when our mind is most reliable, and times when it is less so.

Accepting thoughts at face value or seeing them as permanent can lead to misperceptions. Sometimes, because we think our thoughts are permanent, we try to avoid unpleasant thoughts. Paradoxically, the more we try to avoid thinking of something, the more we end up thinking about it.[37] What if I asked you to close your eyes right now and not think of a pink elephant? It's not so easy, is it? In fact, it's probably hard to think of anything else. Some people, instead of noticing the unpleasant thoughts and uncomfortable feelings or urges that come with them, try to avoid them altogether with behavior.

There are other ways of avoiding discomfort that are not outward behaviors but rather use internal mechanisms. Depressive numbness and rumination have been described as a turning away from life.[38] Though it's often unconscious, it causes us to lose contact with present reality and the natural cycle of life's ups and downs. Post-traumatic stress disorder (PTSD) brings people roaring back into the past with flashbacks. Anxiety disorders keep such a tight focus on the future with what-if scenarios that people can misperceive the true size of a danger that's right in front of them. Attention disorders hijack the mind away from the task at hand, often toward more pleasant daydream states. Impulse disorders temporarily take us away from the present moment and whatever we may find uncomfortable in it. These all become habits of mind, ruts we get into. The power of mindfulness is that it enables us to make contact with the here and now and accept whatever is going on, gracefully parrying the onslaught of these various forms of suffering that take place really only in our imagination. When children are empowered with the knowledge, skill, and wisdom of mindfulness and stay present, they avoid creating much suffering and pain for themselves and those around them. Research has also found that mindfulness and acceptance practices lead to an increased willingness to try more new therapies and take calculated risks. This is important for anxious people and can increase a person's willingness to face their fears, even therapy.

Depression

Free yourself from mental slavery, none but ourselves can free our mind.
—Bob Marley

Rates of depression appear to be rising in both children and adults around the world.[39] Depression is more profound than just sadness; it represents one of the most dangerous mental illnesses, in the most severe cases leading to death by suicide. The most recent estimates suggest that over a lifetime about a quarter of women and half as many men will experience depression, and many of these will experience it as part of bipolar disorder. Though childhood depression is less common, rates for adolescents are similar to those for adults.[40] While the observations of parents, teachers, and other caregivers are an important part of the diagnostic process, consultation with a clinician is the only way to effectively diagnose mood disorders. Feelings of sadness are one symptom of depression, so sadness is often confused with depression because it can feel so uncomfortable. Yet it is important to remember that sadness is an ordinary and universal human emotion that serves important purposes in human experience.

Many treatments already exist for childhood depression. Medication targets the biological factors, and psychotherapy and other lifestyle modifications work with the social and psychological factors.[41] Though medication is a common treatment, it doesn't always help. It's most effective in conjunction with some kind of psychotherapy. Most medications aren't clinically tested on children and the long-term effects of medication on the brain remain unknown. Side effects are common, and young children may not be able to accurately describe them. Psychotherapy and play-and-talk therapies have been used for years and have been shown to be effective in both depressed children and adults.

If treatments exist for childhood depression, what can mindfulness add? Many caregivers are rightfully skeptical of medication—as well as the financial ties that some doctors and researchers have to the pharmaceutical industry—as the only answer. Furthermore, even with treatment, depression comes back. A team of psychologists in Great Britain has recently developed a mindfulness-based treatment for depression (MBCT) in adults that has now been clinically proven to reduce relapse in the chronically depressed by almost half.[42] The program has already been loosely adapted for children by Randye Semple in California. Still other studies have shown mindfulness therapies to reduce depressive symptoms.[43] These promising results suggest that, whether you're a therapist or simply a supportive teacher, parent, or caregiver, incorporating some mindfulness training into your work with depressed children and teens will be helpful to their recovery.

My supervisor, Dr. Stephanie Morgan, describes depression as the numbing and dulling of the experience of life, suppressing our natural vitality and turning us inward and away from life. Mindfulness, as we know, has the opposite effect, bringing us into contact with life, the pains and the joys. Rather than letting the brain numb itself to these pains and joys, or even change them, mindfulness allows us to change our relationship to these experiences of life in an accepting way.

I often suggest with both kids and adults that they think about the "top ten playlists" of negative self-talk that play on repeat. From there, they can learn new songs and sing along to create a new top ten. Another way to deal with the negative thoughts is to repeat them aloud over and over again until they become meaningless, or to have kids practice saying them to themselves, but in funny voices like Daffy Duck or SpongeBob.

Research has also shown that depressed people interpret their experiences more negatively than others and ruminate on them whether they are good, bad, or neutral. This is clearly fuel for the fire of depression.[44] Another study has shown that mindfulness practice reduced the number of negative stories people told themselves. As negative thoughts become less believable and less common, they lose the power to shape reality for a person. Even children who are not depressed but may be suffering from low self-esteem can benefit from exercises that bring awareness to these thoughts and learn to take them with a grain of salt.

My patient, who I will call Rachel, used to feel like a constant failure in her high-pressure high school and became so despairing and full of shame that she literally would not make eye contact for more than a few seconds during the course of a fifty-minute session. She was pretty skeptical about mindfulness practice, but she did agree to step back and observe her thoughts and it seemed to help. First, increased awareness helped Rachel to bring into conscious focus in what situations and how often her negative self-talk thoughts occurred. "Aha, I'm having that 'I'm a failure' thought again that Chris asked me to watch for—it usually happens around studying and also around certain friends." From here, without judgment she was able to understand that she need not accept the thought at face value but rather accept it as just a thought, impermanent and distinct from herself and her reality.

As a strong science student, she could also conceive of it in a way that made sense to her: "This is only a thought created by the circuits in my brain, probably responding to something automatically because of my conditioning, and it's not necessarily the truth at all." With more practice, she was able to have a better perspective on the events in her mind. "I can remember that I, like everyone, have felt like a failure in some situations, maybe even this one, but not necessarily all situations. In fact, failure is only one way of seeing this situation—I can also see it as an opportunity." Over time, Rachel spoke more in our sessions, opening up both to herself and to me about where some of her most self-critical thoughts came from, including echoes from middle school bullies and her parents' pressure on her and for her success.

✻ *Practice 7.1: The Parade of Thoughts*[45]

Invite your child to adopt a comfortable position, gently closing his eyes, bringing his attention first to his breathing and then his thoughts.

Ask him to imagine a big circus-like parade coming down the street. Anything and everything could be in this parade, because this parade is larger than the universe, this parade is the size of your imagination and mind. You can use this script or adapt as fits the situation: Imagine this parade marching outward from the side of your head and circling around in front of your eyes where you can simply sit and watch it unfold, watching what comes next. Everything is in this parade, thoughts, feelings, sensations, some crazy, some boring. With each thought that comes up, you notice someone in the parade holding up a sign, or perhaps there is a sign painted on the side of each float. The sign has your thought written on it, with perhaps a few words or maybe a picture that represents the thought.

Just watch the parade go by, noticing the signs for as long as you can. If you find yourself joining the parade, or if the parade stops, try to bring your attention back to where it had been just before. Put a sign on whatever is marching past and go back to sitting and watching. Remember now that all of your thoughts are just thoughts, part of the parade. When a thought becomes overwhelming, you can put it on a sign and let it march away as it's certain to do eventually.

Allow the child to experiment with this for a moment or two, and try assigning it as homework for even just a few minutes a day. Help the child notice which thoughts consistently stop the parade, and which ones want to grab him or her to join the parade.

Walking Meditation

People usually consider walking on water or in thin air a miracle. But I think the real miracle is not to walk either on water or in thin air, but to walk on earth. Every day we are engaged in a miracle which we don't even recognize: a blue sky, white clouds, green leaves, the black curious eyes of a child—our own two eyes. All is a miracle.
—Thich Nhat Hanh

Another mindfulness activity that can help with mood is walking meditation. One of the basic qualities of depression that people describe is feeling stuck or trapped. The simple act of walking and moving can help someone feel as if she's slowly but surely moving somewhere and at least doing something. Walking, one of the simplest and most basic of human activities, might be better for low-energy depressed children. Studies of mild exercise also have found it to be as effective in helping with depression as therapy or medication—sometimes even more effective.[46] Other studies of mindfulness courses have found that participants report greater enjoyment of exercise, which will in turn help them with their depression. Thich Nhat Hanh and many other teachers recommend mindful walking to serve as a bridge between formal mindfulness practice and mindfulness practice in our daily lives. Kids also do well with physical movement meditations. Indoors, you may choose to walk in a circle around the room, varying the pace to allow different body sensations to arise. Outside, you can walk in larger circles or on a path. During walking, you may also wish to emphasize a particular sensory awareness, such as sounds or smells.

One exercise that I've done with kids in urban areas is to try to bring attention to the life that exists in their concrete world—ants on the sidewalk, green weeds or ivy snaking out of cracks in the cement. Counting the number of breaths in each step can also help maintain focus. Older teens may like to repeat the mantra with each footfall, "No where to go…Nothing to do…no one to be…." Again, adapt the exercise for your children according to their particular context and in ways that they'll respond to. Introducing walking meditation and occasionally practicing it in the hallway is a great exercise for teachers to try with their classes.

* *Practice 7.2: Walking Meditation*[47]

In every walk with nature, one receives far more than he seeks.
—John Muir

Use this script or adapt it to your situation: Long before the arrival of Europeans, thousands of tribes of Native Americans roamed the lands of North and South America. They loved and honored the land that they walked on, and all the creatures that shared their environment. When the children would reach a certain age, they spent some time in the woods to prepare themselves for adulthood. In the silence of the woods, they would come to discover themselves and their place in the world. The silence was necessary so as to not frighten away the creatures of the forest. Silence was necessary to listen to nature. They learned how to walk silently, mindfully through the forest in order to not disturb what was happening around them.

Standing now and smiling, let's try to walk as they did, as quietly and as gently as possible on the earth. With each step, pay close mindful attention to your feet and body. Now gently breathe in, and follow your breath down to the sensations in your legs and feet. We will start by gently lifting our right leg, noticing the sensations as our muscles tense. Then gently begin to lower it. Bring your attention to the bottom of your feet as you gently set your heel down first, and then silently set the rest of your foot and your toes down on to the earth, and feel the weight of your body shifting onto this foot and away from your left foot.

Notice that your body instinctively knows how to walk, how to balance without even having to think about it. Thank your body for its own wisdom. Feel your left heel come back gently to the floor or earth, softly moving the rest of your foot down. When your mind wanders, simply notice where it goes and return to the task at hand. Let the earth hold you; trust your body to carry you along. Walk without a destination, walk just for this step, just for this breath...completely in the moment...notice how silent you can make your footsteps as we walk together.

Bring other senses into the walk as well, and help your students notice their reactions. A burly young man named Antoine who typically talked pretty tough and had a lot of issues with anger described his responses to the walking meditation: "I never noticed how my mood changes just a bit as I walked from a shadow into the sunlight, and how strong the urge was to speed up to get back to the sunlight. And it was crazy when I smelled fresh-cut grass how much I was back to childhood memories of summertime, and feelings, all kinds—good and bad—just flooded over me, it was almost overwhelming when I let myself be open. But what really hit me was how much I was aware of other people looking at us as we mindfully walked down the street." Our mindful walk was very slow and thoughtful. "It was almost too much, the racing thoughts I was having as we walked—"these people think we're crazy, they must think we're in a cult or something, I hope I don't see anyone I know.... On one level I didn't care, but on another I was really, really self-conscious. But after we were back, and I was thinking about it after group, it just hit me how many little thoughts I'm having all day that are changing my mood, and then my behavior. Steering me away from this thing or person and toward this other, bringing up thoughts that change my whole attitude, which is constantly changing and responding all the time without my even knowing it."

Anxiety and Fear

Move outside the tangle of fear-thinking. Live in silence.
—RUMI

I've experienced many terrible events in my life. A few of which actually happened.
—MARK TWAIN

A child was once wandering in the woods on a summer's day. Growing tired, he sat himself down beneath a tree to rest. What he did not realize was that he was sitting under a magical tree that made every thought or desire he had come true. He sat and rested, thinking about how tired he was. "This tree is a nice place to rest," he thought, "but a little house with a bed would certainly be more pleasant." Suddenly—POOF!—there was a cottage right in front of him. He looked in and seeing a comfortable bed and big fluffy pillows, he walked inside and slept for the night.

When he awoke from his rest, he found his stomach growling and he thought, "Oh, I'm so hungry, I wonder if there's any food in this cabin." No sooner did he have the thought than a plate of his favorite food arrived. He ate quickly, and soon was no longer hungry. But he found himself growing impatient. "I wish there was something to do around here," he thought and suddenly he had more games and toys and entertainers than he knew what to do with. He played with the toys a while, watched the performers put on a show, but soon found himself alone and bored again.

At this point, he was starting to think something was a little fishy. "What is this all about?" he wondered. "Whenever I have a thought, it seems to come true. Maybe this tree is haunted. Is there a genie or some other magical creature here?" And a genie appeared. The boy was now quite frightened. "Oh dear, perhaps it's not a friendly genie but a demon in disguise sent here for some reason..." and the genie morphed into a demon, complete with sharp teeth and claws. "Oh my, maybe he's going to eat me!" the boy thought, beginning to panic. And the demon did.[48]

Anxiety disorders are the most common psychological problems among children.[49] Anxiety differs from the normal human response of fear in that it triggers the psychological and physiological fear response in safe situations, creating feelings of danger where there needn't be any. Typically, a suffering child knows this fear is irrational, adding shame and embarrassment to the equation. The anxious child comes to fear that very fear itself and goes to great lengths to avoid any situation that might trigger the response. Worrying, another avoidance strategy, is actually effective in the short term, as it temporarily reduces the physiological symptoms of anxiety. But chronic worry leads to longer-term problems.

Some of the most creative and intelligent adults and children are the ones who suffer from the worst anxiety. A particularly bright or creative child can probably think of hundreds more scenarios that would cause, say, her airplane to crash, than someone not as bright or creative. Mindfulness practice allows one to be aware of the thoughts and bodily sensations that accompany fear as mental events that need not be feared in themselves. They are demons, creations of the mind, which reflect something about genetics and life experience, but that don't necessarily reflect reality. After this awareness, one can start to break away from getting caught up in the story about the plane crash and just notice that the mind creates stories about planes crashing. It's the thought patterns that are the conditions under which the problem thrives. With anxiety, as with depression, mindfulness seeks to change our relationship to thoughts, thereby empowering the individual and disempowering the thoughts. With time, the relationship can become one of befriending fear.[50] At the root, anxiety and stress come from the mind not being in the here and now—they come from worrying about the future, second-guessing the past, or wondering about what's happening somewhere else. Attention to the present gently pulls attention away from anxious places such as past, future, or elsewhere so that we can be more effective in the moment in which we're living. Mindful grounding gently redirects the mind and body back to the present and away from the future and the what-if state of anxiety. We can still observe and consider those what-if scenarios, but we need not let them hijack our mind over and over. Worrying, someone wise once said, is planning more than once. "The goal of mindfulness" one author writes, "is to develop wisdom, to see what is true and to act wisely."[51]

One direct route into the present moment for adults and children is through our senses and the exercises that focus present moment awareness on sounds, sensations, sights, or smells. Once we are back in the present, we are away from the anxiety.

* *Practice 7.3: Mindful Grounding Words*

My co-worker Stacy has an elementary-school-aged daughter who becomes easily overwhelmed and anxious in unfamiliar situations; her mind becomes frozen in her fears about the future and she starts to unravel. The family came up with an exercise to bring her back in touch with the present through focusing on her body in the present rather than getting stuck in her mind or the future. Stacy or her husband stands behind their daughter and draw letters or spell words on her back with their fingers, gathering and transferring her attention to sensations in the present moment as well as evoking feelings of comfort and support from her loving mom and dad, as they write reminders of her own strengths in the words they choose.

*

Guided Visualizations

Another colleague of mine, Rhonda, used the exercise below to help her son prepare for his cello audition by visualizing Yo-Yo Ma, and many children enjoy this visualization to help them prepare for sports or music tryouts, or for any situation in which they're going to be asked to perform. The reality rarely turns out to be as frightening as we make it in our mind.

Guided visualizations are a different form of meditation that many of us in the West are more familiar with, though they have a long tradition in Tibet and other parts of the world as well. Such meditation exercises can empower children in relation to their fears, while helping them with a particular skill or places they get stuck or anxious. It would make sense that visualizations would assist with planning, practice, and even with performance of certain activities that may be difficult. I've also had positive experiences doing athletic visualizations with children as an introduction to other meditative practices.

✻ *Practice 7.4 : The Maestro*[52]

First, help the child relax and feel comfortable, either sitting or lying down. Begin with another relaxation technique or with focusing on the breath. Once the child is relaxed, begin guiding her through the exercise called the master, maestro, or dream coach. This is one that can be done in either a group or individually. Use this script and shorten or adapt as fits: Imagine now that you are alone, and preparing to practice your favorite game, activity, sport, or instrument. You are the only person in the concert hall or stadium, and you are just there to practice and perfect your art. You can feel your hands on the surface of the ball, racket, or instrument, and even smell the scents that you think of. Just let yourself practice for a moment.

As you are feeling increasingly confident and ready, you can hear footsteps echoing in the distance. You hold that feeling of confidence, and looking into the distance in the hall or arena, you can make out your hero, the role model whom you aspire to play. He or she approaches and smiles at you. You smile back, perhaps surprised at how friendly this person is, this master of the art. The master teacher approaches you and offers to help you with whatever aspect or aspects of your art you want the most help. Just take a few minutes now to listen to the master artist, hear advice, and learn to move as the master does.

Take a few minutes to let the child work with the "master."

Now, keeping in mind the master's lessons, try to visualize your own body moving with the skills that you just learned. Your abilities are just that much better than before, just that much closer to perfect, and the master compliments you on your hard work. It is time to leave now, but the master reminds you that he is always there to talk to you and help you when you are practicing. You can always hear the master's voice by listening deeply within your body. Perhaps you want to thank the master, and watch him or her depart, with the master's voice still ringing in your mind, and the new skills still vibrating in your muscles. Let your mind and body simply remember your lesson for a while. And now, keeping the feeling with you, just wiggle your toes a little bit, and your fingertips, and feel your eyes open. Now take just a moment to practice your skills with your physical body. Allow about a minute, then suggest they mentally rehearse for another minute, then with their body once more.

Body Awareness

Body awareness is helpful in the moment of anxiety, and on a daily basis helps reset the anxiety threshold and helps people come to be preventatively aware of their body's warning systems. Body scans and similar awareness practices are an excellent way to create a mindful awareness of the interconnection of body and mind. These help the person identify where anxieties arise in the body and become aware of the connection of sensations to thoughts and feelings.

* *Practice 7.5: Body Scan*[53]

Find a comfortable place to sit or lie for an extended period of time. Ask your child or the group of children you are working with to notice or measure how stressed their bodies and minds feel before they start, maybe offering a number from one to ten, or perhaps taking their own pulse. Another variation is to have children trace the outlines of their bodies and write or draw, or even just use colors to show where in their bodies they feel emotions, memories, thoughts, and other sensations after the body scan.

Script: Move your body into a comfortable position. Allow the floor or chair to hold you, trusting your body to breathe for you as you bring your awareness to your breath. As you breathe in, let your consciousness flow into and through your body, noticing the body's various points of contact with the floor or cushions. Now bringing your awareness to your breath, follow your breath deep into your body, imagining it reaching all the way down into your legs and feet, shining a flashlight on all of the sensations there. Bring your awareness into your toes, just noticing any sensations there. Be aware of temperature, the sensation of socks if you're wearing socks, your skin and any feeling in the muscles and bones. Now, aware of your breath again, follow your breath into your feet, aware of any other sensations in your feet. Take a moment just to be with your feet and notice how they feel. Your feet have been carrying you around all day. You may want to thank them for their hard work. Breathing again, follow your breath into your ankles. Again, just notice any sensations in your ankles, and what thoughts might come up when you notice the feelings. Breathe now into your lower legs, shining the light on any sensations there. Are they positive, negative, neutral? Do the sensations change or are they constant? Perhaps they throb or come and go in waves? Relax your lower legs? Breathe into your knees, noticing sensations and what thoughts arise with each sensation. Do you want the feeling to end, to continue? Now breathe into your thighs, noticing anything happening from your skin on into your muscle and down into your bones. Are there any urges to move or change position? Now breathe in and bring your awareness to your hips, to any sensations in your hips, and notice the thoughts that arise with the sensations. When your attention naturally wanders, gently note where it has gone and bring your awareness back to your body. Slowly breathing in, follow the air to your abdomen. Be aware of any movement as your belly expands and contracts. Now follow the breath into your chest and your lower back, shining the light here on sensations and thoughts and feelings that you notice. Now breathe into the upper back and shoulders. If worries are in your shoulders, give them a break, let them go free, carried away on the breath. Gently breathe into the fingertips and hands, bringing warm healing air into the hands...aware of any sensations. Now into the wrists and forearms....Breathe in now to your upper arms and shoulders, aware of the sensations in this part of the body and your response to those sensations. When the mind wanders, which it will, observe where it goes and bring it back to the present moment, back to your body. Now breathe into your neck, feeling your muscles and what they are telling you. Breathe again, following that breath into the back of your head, aware of how your head feels, and now into the front of your head and your face. Just notice sensations as they arise, noticing thoughts and feelings that go with them, noticing them fade away or change over time. Notice your mind's response to your body and breathe with it, welcoming it like an old friend. And take a moment now to thank the parts of your body for their hard work—your feet and legs for carrying you, your arms for working to lift things, your chest and all the organs in your torso working hard to pump blood, digest, breathe and keep you alive, and your head and mind and your senses as well.

Pause and breathe.

Slowly return your attention from the inside of your body to the outside and to the room around you. Feeling the safe and soft cushion beneath you, your clothes against your skin, allowing your eyes to gently open, taking with you into the rest of the day this new awareness and friendship with your body.

Ask the children what sensations they noted: you may even want to make a list—itchy, sore, relaxed, throbbing, tense, loose, tingly, heavy, and other such words, seeing who experienced what, and how many things they felt.

---

*

Gabriel, a man I worked with once in a halfway house, had an old injury in his knee that always bothered him and he used this exercise very effectively. The old injury was preventing him from being more active and often served as a trigger for him to relapse with alcohol. Gabriel was in his mid-forties, though the way he walked around stooped over in pain he looked years older. He found the body scan relaxing, though he was initially reluctant to pay more attention to the pain in his body. With some encouragement, he gave it a try and found at first that breathing into his knee seemed to relieve the pain. Over time, however, he came back reporting that it had stopped "working," a lesson in impermanence and attachment to outcomes. I encouraged him to keep trying, and to let go of the expectation that it would work or not work but just to watch what happened.

Gabriel tried again and reported back that he was noticing that the "pain" that he was experiencing was impermanent. "It's not actually always there, I just tell myself it is. It changes—sometimes it pulses, and sometimes it's more of an uncomfortable tickle than it is a sharp pain, but there are always gaps, always moments that it's not there." What had always been present for Gabriel was the story he told himself and the self-pity that accompanied it more than the pain itself. Now the story was starting to fade away. The pain remained the pain, but the suffering lifted as he let go of the story that was creating more anxiety about the pain and leading him into relapse after relapse. As his pain lifted somewhat, and he stayed sober for longer, his posture and the way he carried himself seemed to shift as well, and he actually began to look closer to his age.

Transforming Psychological Trauma

The tears I shed yesterday have become rain.
—Thich Nhat Hanh

Trauma is a tragic and all-too-common event in the lives of the many child survivors around the globe. Though trauma has become more clearly understood in our wider culture, we still often think of a trauma as only one horrifying event, like physical or sexual abuse. We can forget that traumas can be emotional, or can be an ongoing event like neglect. Trauma can include the death or sickness of a friend or classmate, a family member or pet, even a chronic illness in the child. Other traumas include surviving natural disasters like hurricanes or tsunamis, and man-made disasters that range from car accidents to war, to the chronic trauma of poverty and oppression.

Children, whose brains are still developing, are particularly at risk for trauma reactions and often have a lower threshold for processing trauma than adults. At the same time, however, the plasticity of the child's mind, especially when practicing mindfulness, may make recovery more rapid than for adults. Daniel Siegel writes in his book *The Mindful Brain*, "In mindfulness we direct our attention to our intention. Where attention goes, neurons fire. And where neurons fire, they can rewire."

Perhaps the best-known consequence of trauma is post-traumatic stress disorder, PTSD. It is estimated that over a lifetime, PTSD will affect one in ten women, and slightly fewer men.[54] Though not everyone who survives a trauma develops classic PTSD, eight percent do. Others may develop some of the PTSD symptoms or go on to develop different full-blown psychological disorders or interpersonal problems that are rooted in the original trauma. These may include anxiety, depression, other "dissociative" disorders, suicidal behavior, substance abuse, rage, mood swings, and self-injury like cutting.[55]

As disturbing as these are, each of these reactions is, in its own way, understandable as a survival mechanism to deal with the horror of the initial trauma. I've even asked older patients how their behaviors enabled them to survive. Answers were devastatingly truthful and to the point: "the physical pain of cutting blocked my emotional pain"; "depression kept me safe in bed—it sheltered me from the world"; "anger kept others at a safe distance." Children often manifest their trauma reactions differently than adults, often by acting out rather than using their words. Frequently they engage in repetitive and reenacting play, forever stuck trying to resolve what happened. Other children may struggle with behaviors ranging from attention issues to aggression problems.

Trauma experts describe three types of PTSD symptoms: re-experiencing, avoidance, and arousal. Re-experiencing can include invasive memories and flashbacks, nightmares, or reactions to internal and external triggers. Avoidance can include staying away from thoughts, feelings, people, or places that have been mentally linked with the event, as well as a restricted range of emotion. Arousal may include difficulty with sleeping or concentrating as well as hypervigilance.[56] Mindfulness and mindful grounding activities can mitigate all three of these. Typically trauma should be processed through slow-paced long-term therapy. Learning to tolerate the frightening and overwhelming feelings that come up when the event is remembered and building skills for putting the memories away are a major part of treatment.

Grounding exercises are helpful for all forms of anxiety but particularly with trauma. I've had great success with people both practicing and really enjoying this variation on other sense awareness exercises. As a too-cool twelve year old once told me, "Counting to ten when you're upset is played out." So this variation on counting to ten is simple and adds a mindfulness dimension.

✱ *Practice 7.6: Counting to Your Senses*

Count to five in all your senses as you're walking. For younger children, you can count to three. To begin, count five sounds that you hear (this can include your own breathing). Then count five things that you see. To make it more challenging, or for older children, you can add another restriction, for example, count five things you see of the same color, or five round things, or five things made out of wood. Next count five things that you can touch, and then five things that you can smell. Smell and taste will be the harder ones, so allow some leeway. Children can taste the air, their skin, perhaps drink some water, or notice the taste sensations that already exist in their mouth (their teeth, roof of the mouth, etc.).

✱

Jill, a girl in middle school who I worked with for some time, had major anxiety that arose after her parents' contentious divorce. The trauma had reset her baseline anxiety, first leaving her hypervigilant in school and building to create a major school-phobia after she had a panic attack in the cafeteria. She was brightly optimistic in spite of her anxiety, always bubbly and bouncing in her pink hoodie and coke-bottle glasses. She practiced counting to her senses on the walk to school and then in the building and reported with excitement her growing confidence about going to school. Gradually her anxiety waned, and it was almost as if you could see the tension in her body unwinding over time, though certain things would wind her back up again.

"I was walking to school and counting my senses and just the sounds was calming me down. When I got to counting sensations, I noticed that my heartbeat was speeding up again, and at first I worried that I was going to freak out and have another panic attack. But I kept going with my senses and by the time I got back to my body sensations my heart had slowed down again and I wasn't as afraid." Plus, as she pointed out another time, she really enjoyed and appreciated everything that was happening in the world around her that she might never have noticed if she were stuck in her worrying mind about whether she was going to panic in school. If she had needed to, she could have even mixed in some deep breathing or another calming practice once she noticed her heart speeding up. Jill's panic attacks subsided, her school-phobia started to decrease, and eventually she was able to talk more about her feelings about her parents without becoming so emotional.

All manners of trauma can be soothed by meditation practices, which allow space for the internal and external rebuilding that needs to happen to be able to live with trauma. One powerful study examined villagers in the aftermath of a cyclone in Bangladesh some years ago. The researchers found that the villagers with meditative traditions recovered faster from the trauma of the disaster and had lower rates of post-traumatic stress. When I was recently in Dharamsala, the seat of the Tibetan Government-in-Exile, I met a number of monks who had escaped across the Himalayas to find freedom in India. The survivors credited their meditation practice with enabling them not just to withstand the torture and horror they had endured as political prisoners in their own country, but to give them resilience to avoid developing many PTSD symptoms that would have haunted other survivors.

So how does mindfulness help with trauma? Mindfulness increases thought *awareness*. This allows the practitioner to notice patterns of thought that may be related to trauma. This includes thought triggers, the content of our thoughts, and our emotional reactions to those thoughts, such as Jill's noticing her body getting activated and then soothing herself. For the traumatized person or child, this awareness is healing on a number of levels. First, seeing the frightening patterns as they are—thoughts from the past, not reality in the present—is itself empowering and liberating. This insight leads to responding to the present event rather than to the past trauma. For the traumatized child whose thoughts may carry him or her away to unpleasant or "dissociated" places, mindful awareness of thoughts allows the child to catch himself earlier, before he's carried into the stream of thought and finds himself drowning. In this way, mindful grounding practices can work as a psychological life preserver, helping people pull themselves to safety.

A mindful emphasis on the present moment, here and now, alleviates trauma-related symptoms as well.[57] Remaining safely in touch with the present reality forestalls the "re-experiencing" of dissociation and flashbacks or the urge to avoid them through behavior. Many of the traumatic symptoms include the invasion of events from the past and elsewhere into the present. The problematic behaviors often seen in adult and child trauma survivors (mistrust, explosive anger, substance abuse, and other avoidance strategies) arise from well-intentioned attempts to keep those flashbacks or emotions at bay—and they work, they just have other consequences. With a focus on the here and now, on this moment, thoughts and actions are neither distracted nor dictated by the past. The survivor becomes attuned to the truth of the moment instead of being over-attuned to possible danger, and so can respond from a menu of choices rather than an unconscious reaction.

The so-called arousal symptoms of PTSD, such as loss of concentration, sleep difficulties, and hyperarousal, are also all naturally aided by meditation's calming effects on the mind and body.[58] Meditation can decrease the constant hyperarousal of brain and body and help regulate emotions. Studies with trauma survivors have found that meditation and mindfulness practices helped them learn to better anticipate, identify, and tolerate emotionally charged thoughts, feelings, and memories. Other studies show mindfulness practice aids recovery from stress and boosts resilience before a trauma occurs.[59]

Below, I've adapted a mindful grounding exercise utilized by trauma experts who treat combat veterans in Israel.

✻ *Practice 7.7: Four Elements Story and Meditation*

There are four elements that can help us find a moment of peace, a moment of grounding, and a moment of healing. If we plant the seed now, we can grow peace in ourselves, and nurture it in our communities until there is peace in the world.

Stand up like a tree rooted in the ground, blossoming in the desert. Close your eyes if you feel comfortable, or keep them open with your gaze a little bit in front of you on the floor if that feels safer. We will take strength from the four ancient elements we're made of: earth, air, water, and fire. First we ground ourselves, aware of where we are and where we stand on this Earth. Feel your feet firmly planted on the floor, their roots going down into the earth. Imagine yourself like a desert tree, rooted, unmoving in the desert and blossoming in spite of your surroundings. Gently keep a small smile on your lips. Now, as you breathe in through your nose, be aware of the air in the room, its smell and taste. This is the same air that everyone breathes, our friends and our enemies, the same air we all breathe all across the world and across the centuries, the same air that our ancestors breathed, that even the dinosaurs breathed. We share this life-giving air with countless other beings. This is the breath of life, we breathe and we know we are alive. Next, be aware of water, another element we must have for life to be possible. Swallow the saliva in your mouth, aware of your jaw, tongue, and other muscles working, and feel it naturally following its path downward. Finally, be aware of the fire of life in our bellies and minds. Notice the thoughts dancing in our heads that make us alive and human.

✻

Autism and Asperger's

I'm asked often whether these practices can be helpful for children with autism or Asperger's. This is not an area in which a lot of research has been done, but logic would say that they could. As I mentioned earlier, Paul Fulton describes mindfulness practice as a form of universal exposure therapy, and for many children with spectrum-related cognitive styles, developing a capacity for sensory tolerance is both incredibly difficult and incredibly important. A relaxed state can help a child learn to tolerate small amounts of difficult sensory input or eye contact without becoming too aroused or anxious. These practices can bypass verbal mediation and go straight to a deeper level of processing and change.

8

Practices for Positive Choices

Between thought and expression lies a lifetime.
—Lou Reed

Patience in a moment of anger will save one hundred days of tears.
—Khmer Proverb

A traditional West African folktale goes like this: Many years ago, there was a village that grew the juiciest mangos around. Because they were so delicious, people from all over the continent sought out these mangos and traded for them. One year, the villagers went to harvest their mangos and found that they were gone. They heard something and looked into the leaves of the trees where they saw monkeys laughing as they ate the mangos of the villagers. One of the old wise men in the village remembered a time long past when monkeys had caused trouble. The villagers had designed a trap from a hollowed out coconut into which they drilled a hole wide enough for a monkey's arm to enter, but too small for it to come out once it had made a fist. In the center of the trap they placed a fruit as bait. Eventually a monkey would come by, smell the mango, and reach his arm into the trap. As soon as he grasped the mango, he made a tight fist and tried to pull his arm back out. But to no avail—the monkey pulled and pulled, but his fist was too big to come out of the hole in the trap. Of course, the monkey could get his arm out, but he would have to first unclasp his fist. Here was the monkey—trapped because he had grasped what he wanted in the moment, but he was unable to see that what had worked to get him what he wanted in the moment was unable to bring him what he truly desired or needed in the long-term. The villagers would simply pick the monkey up, his fist still tight inside the trap, and walk him far from the village where he wouldn't disturb them.

This story is a perfect example of impulse control. Letting go of the impulse is the key to getting out of the trap—the trap that works to get us what we want in the moment but not the long term. Otherwise, what we want is within our grasp, but never truly ours.

Many grown-ups and young people avoid emotional discomfort by resorting to impulse problems: cutting, hitting, addictions, eating disorders, explosive anger, and other behaviors that relieve the discomfort in the moment but lead to greater suffering in the long run. Freud and the Buddha each described versions of what's been dubbed the pleasure principle. This is the simple idea that says we naturally seek the pleasurable and avoid the painful or unpleasant, and that we suffer from this constant grasping and aversion. The flip side of avoiding psychological discomfort is seeking psychological pleasure, mistaking pleasure for happiness. We as humans unconsciously get into routines that seek fleetingly pleasurable states of mind rather than observing and accepting pleasure as impermanent and happiness as a separate entity altogether. We think of children in particular as having difficulty delaying gratification, yet we adults are often no better. Meditative practices have been well-proven by history and now by research to have a powerful effect on regulating strong emotions and suppressing impulses long enough to make different choices and in turn reducing those self-destructive behaviors.[60]

Strong urges and impulses are hard for any of us to control, but they are especially hard for young people who often have not fully developed their prefrontal cortex. Our bodies naturally create impulses to act, and in an evolutionary sense this is in the interest of our safety. Imagine if we took the time to consciously think before responding to a saber-toothed tiger leaping out at us instead of just diving out of the way. But in our safer world today, we often need to respond more slowly and carefully through thinking and planning, or what neuropsychologists call executive functioning.

No one turns to self-destructive behaviors just to worry people or rebel. They turn to them because they work—they are very effective at changing how we feel, a process that holds true at the neural level as well. Many of these impulsive behaviors are more efficient than prescription drugs (or even street drugs) in changing our emotional state. Brain research has even shown that self-cutting releases powerful euphoria-inducing chemicals in the brain, as well as the empowering rush of adrenaline and endorphins. For some people, compulsive shopping, stealing, or gambling has the same biochemical rush. It's no wonder people give in to these impulses, and no wonder it becomes as hard to stop as any chemical addiction. The problem is that while such behaviors may change the feelings temporarily, the long-term consequences—like with addiction—typically get worse and worse. This also makes suggesting mindfulness practices difficult.

A short mindfulness exercise hardly works as quickly or powerfully as giving into the impulse to cut, get high, punch a wall, shoplift, or engage in another problematic behavior. When I speak with teens about their behavior, I simply try to be as honest about this as possible, by validating their reasons. "From what you are telling me, your behavior has been getting you into trouble. On the other hand, it works to get rid of the really bad feelings that can just completely take over sometimes, and so I can understand. I have another idea for you. It may not work as quickly or completely as your behavior has, but it does help a little bit and it doesn't have the same negative consequences. If punching the wall works as a ten out of ten, mindfulness is maybe a two. But later, mindfulness is a zero for consequences, and punching the wall means a bruised or cut hand, and feeling shame."

Kids, particularly teenagers, appreciate this straightforward talk. But we can't just suppress an impulse, we have to suggest where it should go. When it comes to changing behaviors, we cannot just block off the highway exit, we must also be responsible for clearly marking where the detour goes. With more options comes freedom, or what I like to call creative empowerment.

If the behavior is not too dangerous or too automatic, I'll sometimes be a bit paradoxical and suggest, "Go ahead and do that, but I'm going to ask you to wait for one minute first, to see how you feel in that minute, and then make the choice to punch that wall, maybe even saying it aloud, and then to make the choice to notice how you feel an hour afterward." With older people who are concerned about their substance abuse, I'll suggest, "I'm not going to tell you not to drink after work on Friday, but I am just going to ask you to wait five minutes before you drink and notice how it feels to not drink, and then you can go ahead and deliberately make the choice to have a drink, come back and tell me a bit about those five minutes." This is what teacher Joseph Goldstein calls the "about to" moment, the time between thought and action when anything can happen if we are aware.

Often people are surprised by the discomfort and become curious about it and gradually learn to tolerate it. Of course, accepting any behaviors requires good judgment of safety and risk on your part, as well as some radical acceptance of the behavior.

One exercise I offer to people who are working on impulse issues is called the CALM reminder. It's essentially a quick body scan and self check-in about any urges.

* *Practice 8.1: Calming Impulses*

First, standing or sitting up straight, bring attention to your breath. Now starting with *C* for chest, breathe relaxation into your chest and allow your heart and lungs to expand and open for a few breaths. Next, bringing awareness to *A*—your arms' sensations, urges, associations for a few calming breaths. And now, shift your attention to *L* for your legs, feeling grounded on the floor and strong, and aware of what comes up in terms of impulses to move, and sit another moment with these. Next, bring attention to *M* for your mind, taking a few breaths to allow the mind to settle further. Check in again with your impulses, and see if you can make a different choice.

———— *

Alice, a young woman I worked with, had a terrible problem with using substances, acting out sexually, and cutting and burning herself. She was scarred up and down her arms, and that was just what I could see. I knew she had more scars hidden, and more emotional scars than

I could imagine. She couldn't control her urges to cut. Even after she had gotten her sex addiction and drug behaviors mostly under control, she would still scratch at herself with a plastic knife or untwisted paper clip.

The only thing that helped her get through to the other side and stop cutting was when she was able to pay attention to her experience a few minutes at a time. Peering through the black bangs that often covered her face, she told me, "I would be feeling terrible and know that I was going to cut and not want to stop, nothing would stop me, so I'd decide okay, I'll cut, no one will stop me, but I'll do it in five minutes, and then sometimes wait another five minutes and another and another and try to sit with it until it passed, or sometimes until it was dinnertime or I had to use the bathroom. What I've realized is that there is just pain. Sometimes that pain does not go away when you want it to, and it kind of definitely doesn't go away when you try to make it go away. It's like a mosquito bite; if you itch it, it goes away for a second and then comes back even stronger.

"So sometimes pain is pain, and there is no making it go away, we just can't. The only power we really can have is to make it worse in the long run, with drugs or cutting or doing something else dumb. So it's almost as if what it comes down to is that pain of life is something we have no power to make better, we only have the power to NOT make it worse. That was kind of depressing at first, but now it's kind of comforting to know what power I have, and what power I don't have."

With some patients, I use the example of an infant. As infants, when we had the impulse to go to the bathroom, we simply went. As we grew older, our parents, on strict orders from society, trained us to notice our impulses and make a plan for how to deal with them appropriately. Now when we get an urge, we are generally able to plan the appropriate steps to avoid creating a mess that would instantly keep people from wanting to have anything to do with us. Unlike toilet training, we do not always receive instructions from parents or society on what to do with emotional impulses and how to handle them in productive ways. Annie, a young woman with substance abuse problems, is someone I worked with for a long time. She still jokes about this metaphor, and yet shares it now with other young women she sponsors in Alcoholics Anonymous (AA).

Children, and teens in particular, make emotional messes by giving in to urges to become explosively angry, use drugs, or cut themselves in order to find relief, leaving those around them to deal with the aftermath. Some do not know how to deal with such impulses as blurting out answers in class, while others can't handle emotional impulses in healthy ways. Giving in to impulses can cause a mess that pushes people away and that no one wants to clean up. It's not easy to tolerate the discomfort that arises when the momentum of our bodies or minds sends a signal to act, but we need to slow down to make a plan. Research is showing more and more that teens and children have a particularly hard time suppressing impulses, and our culture is not doing a great job of teaching them how to do this as they grow older. Mindfulness practice and other skill training can play an important role in helping the child learn tolerance and even compassion for the impulses and offer her a chance to make and implement a skillful plan. Mindfulness creates choices; we may keep ending up in the same restaurant, but we can ask for a menu of responses to choose from rather than just having our regular waiter bring us "the usual," with all its complicated consequences.

So, just like the rest of us, kids can get stuck in these impulsive behaviors that work in the moment but turn out to be traps in the long-term if they keep at them. Fortunately, children are young and their habits are not as entrenched as those of adults.

Noah Levine, a meditation teacher who has worked in juvenile detention facilities with troubled adolescents, adapted the traditional concept of the twelve *nidana*s (causes or origins) of dependent origination from Buddhist psychology to describe the process of giving in to impulses. Here is the chain of thought, feeling, and action Levine describes:

1. Ignorance, which leads to
2. Mental formations (thoughts or emotions), which lead to
3. Consciousness, which requires
4. Material form, which has
5. Six senses (physical sensation, hearing, seeing, smelling, tasting, and mental thoughts) through which stimuli generate
6. Contact, which creates sense impressions that generate

7. Feelings (pleasant, unpleasant, or neutral) that generate
8. Craving (either to keep or to get rid of the feeling), which causes
9. Grasping (or aversion), which generates
10. Becoming (identifying with the experience as personal), which generates
11. Birth (incarnating around the grasping), which generates
12. Suffering or dissatisfaction

Let's look at an example of that sequence in action, in this case, the action of wanting ice cream.

1. I am walking down the street, not paying attention. (Ignorance)
2. I see an ice cream shop, and the thought arises, "Ice cream is delicious and makes me happy." (Mental formation)
3. I decide that I will have some ice cream. (Consciousness)
4. I walk into the ice cream shop. (Material form, my body)
5. Inside the shop, I see and smell the ice cream and begin to think about what kind I shall order. (Senses)
6. The ice cream smells sweet and creamy. (Contact)
7. I enjoy the smells of the waffle cone and hot fudge. (Feelings, pleasant)
8. I decide that I need a triple-scoop hot-fudge sundae in an extra-large waffle cone. (Craving)
9. After a few bites I am full, but I continue to eat the whole thing because it tastes so good. (Grasping at pleasure)
10. I wish I hadn't eaten the whole thing, or had any ice cream at all. I think I was stupid for eating it. (Becoming)
11. I blame myself for being so gluttonous. (Birth)
12. I feel physically sick and emotionally drained. (Suffering)

When it comes to our basic urges, mindfulness operates between the links in the chain, breaking their automatically linking nature with conscious awareness between feeling and craving.[61] A cognitive psychologist might say that this is roughly analogous to breaking the chain of thought and action in cognitive behavioral therapy. The ice cream is one trigger, but other emotional events set off or disrupt the chain at another point. With attention, we can do some "urge surfing," just noticing where in the body and mind urges to act arise. One way to help with this impulsivity and restlessness is this "boredom meditation," adapted from tai chi.

✻ *Practice 8.2: Boredom and Impulse Meditation*

This is a practical and portable exercise that can be done at almost any time. It is easy enough to teach to children, and can be practiced together when waiting around or anywhere that you might tend to get bored. In tai chi, qigong, and other movement meditations, one focuses on moving one's *qi*, a form of energy, through the body. One can fill and empty one's legs of this energy by slowly and carefully shifting weight between the two legs.

Standing about hips width apart or slightly more, find your *dan-tien*, or center point, about three finger widths below your belly button. Breathe into that point for a few breaths, until you feel comfortable with knowing where it is. Feeling your feet rooted in the earth beneath you, slowly move by pushing on the soles of your feet rather than your mind, shifting your dan-tien toward the right, imagining your qi, like water, is pouring into your left leg and filling it as the height of your two hips changes. Your body or mind may want to move more quickly, but imagine you are very carefully pouring the qi in a thin stream into the other leg. Eventually, your left leg will fill with the qi from your right leg when the left foot has no more weight on it. Now, focusing again on the dan-tien, gently move it toward the left, feeling the qi flowing downward and emptying from your left leg into the right leg. Without rushing, focus on the sensations of the energy flowing from leg to leg, seeing how slowly you can pour, how gentle a stream you can make a few drops at a time. Take care to balance your legs and body. Notice and observe any desire or urge to move more quickly, and gently return your attention to pouring the qi into the other leg.

After even a few times of pouring the qi back and forth, you'll find yourself at the front of that line, or at least some of that boredom or impatience relieved for a more settled mind and body.

I'll end this chapter with a poem by Portia Nelson that many of the young people I work with have found helpful in recovering from destructive behaviors.

AUTOBIOGRAPHY IN FIVE SHORT CHAPTERS
Portia Nelson

Chapter I
I walk down the street.
There is a deep hole in the sidewalk.
I fall in.
I am lost...I am helpless.
It isn't my fault.
It takes forever to find a way out.

Chapter II
I walk down the same street.
There is a deep hole in the sidewalk.
I pretend I don't see it.
I fall in again.
I can't believe I am in the same place.
But, it isn't my fault.
It still takes a long time to get out.

Chapter III
I walk down the same street.
There is a deep hole in the sidewalk.
I see it is there.
I still fall in . . . it's a habit.
My eyes are open.
I know where I am.

It is my fault.
I get out immediately.

Chapter IV
I walk down the same street.
There is a deep hole in the sidewalk.
I walk around it.

Chapter V
I walk down another street.

CONCLUSION: Growing a Forest

One generation plants the trees; another gets the shade.
—CHINESE PROVERB

OUR CHILDREN are suffering, as are we and our planet. Even a cursory glance at the news could cause any of us to worry about the present and future. It is easy to become overwhelmed with fears about what kind of world will be left to our children and grandchildren. Environmental devastation, widening gaps between haves and have-nots, disease, war, and human cruelty seem pervasive. We continue, not because things naturally work out, but because in every generation people have worked to make things better. We can choose to pass on practices of liberation or, if we choose not to, we will be passing on practices of suffering.

What inspires me to continue to teach mindfulness and to believe in its effectiveness is the children I work with. When I start to feel burned out I think about Eana, a teenager who stopped speaking after a friend's death and who has now learned to take three deep breaths and then respond to direct questions, allowing her beautiful deep brown eyes to make contact with others for a second at a time. I think of my friend Ryan, who was addicted to a series of drugs since he was an adolescent, who now sits in meditation every morning and evening for ten minutes to create a space between impulse and action. I think of Rachel, who used to believe all the negative stories the bullies in her mind would tell her and how sitting in mindfulness has helped her turn those bullies' shouts into whispers until they became almost completely silent. I saw her crossing the street recently and she carried herself as if she no longer had those bullies whispering into her ear.

When I'm struggling to focus at the end of a long day I think of Ben, a ten-year-old with ADHD and an amazing capacity for both creativity and chaos. Now, using concentration and visualization meditations, he can tell his distraction demons they have to leave him alone for a few minutes while he focuses on his multiplication tables. I still recall the day that Alice, now with bright tattoos covering some of her scars, realized how much power she had to stay away from self-destructive behaviors like cutting. Her self-awareness made her seem as wise as an old Buddhist master! I can imagine Carrie, who was once so helpless that even with an army of hired assistants, she couldn't get through a day without collapsing. Now she leads mindfulness exercises for her hockey team, teaching them to notice sensations in their bodies and the thoughts that come up with them. I will always be grateful to Jeffrey, with ice cream stains on his shirt, for smiling as he reminds me to take my three deep breaths before I roll the dice. I think about the choices that Shane made that led to him sitting in prison for the next fifteen years, but also the liberation that he found there from the seed that was planted by one yoga teacher years ago, a seed he has nurtured and helped grow in extremely harsh and cruel conditions.

I think back to that day on the lake looking at clouds with my father, my first lesson in the power of breathing and an understanding of impermanence. As a teenager and young adult, I forgot this lesson as I struggled with my own anger and sense of direction. Now I have the great privilege of planting seeds of mindfulness in others. When we plant seeds in others, we nurture them in ourselves. Those who spend time with young people already know the blessings of seeing the world through their eyes, and those who teach know how much teaching deepens our own understanding.

In the Hindu legends, there is a concept called *leela*, the play of the cosmos. It was this divine play that created our universe. Working with children puts us in touch with our most playful and creative selves, our best selves. I hope this book helps you plant seeds of mindfulness and compassion in the next generation and, in doing so, awakens your own playful and joyful child's mind.

Appendix 1: Lesson Plans

Never doubt that a small group of thoughtful, committed citizens can change the world. Indeed, it is the only thing that ever has.
—Margaret Mead

The lessons here are intended as a resource for any adults who work with young people in groups and may have the opportunity to do a longer-term group. They are based on the pioneering work of Jon Kabat-Zinn's Mindfulness Based Stress Reduction program. Adaptations of Kabat-Zinn's work have been made for depression and various other disorders. The work of Randye Semple, Daniel Siegel, and Susan Kaiser Greenland is also being tested with children and getting impressive results. Here are some ideas about ways to use the technology that the next generation is fluent in to engage and support their practice.

Each group I've outlined is five sessions and can repeat itself regularly, adding new members and reinforcing content for existing members. These groups are also just suggestions for getting started; there are so many wonderful exercises in this book and elsewhere to consider doing and integrating into your group. Think about what values you want to emphasize with your kids, and make a list. Study the tips recommended earlier in this book and ask others for help, and adapt the practices here and elsewhere to suit you and your situation. You may also want to pick out quotes and stories from this or other books to open and close each group.

Start each week by checking in about the homework, and checking in and out about how people feel in their bodies and minds, maybe using numbers. Ask about what exercises people liked in the previous week, and what experiences with mindfulness people had during the week.

Children's Group (up to age 12)

Outline 1: Basics of Mindful Awareness

OBJECTIVES & KEY POINTS:

- Review expectations and purposes of the group
- Introduce basic elements of mindful awareness through eating and touch
- Pay close attention to things with our senses brings unexpected awareness about them
- Discover how interconnected we are to everyone and everything
- Change the way we breathe can change the way we feel

MATERIALS:

- Basket of oranges or tangerines
- A number of small objects—pinecones, stones, coins, pencils, toys, etc.

ACTIVITIES:

- Know Your Orange, 10 minutes (p. 36) combined with Mindful Eating 10 minutes
- The Six Senses, 15 minutes (p. 48)
- Diaphragmatic or Belly Breathing, 5 minutes (p. 66)

HOMEWORK:

- Three diaphragmatic breaths morning and night

Outline 2: Acceptance and Body Awareness

OBJECTIVES & KEY POINTS:

- Shift perspectives about "good" and "bad," acceptance, looking for the positive

Increase body awareness and relaxation
Notice the impermanence of physical sensations and mental interpretations of the physical

MATERIALS:
Paper and pencils, drawing materials, large roll of paper or smaller pieces of paper

ACTIVITIES:
Sai and the Horse, 15 minutes (p. 64)
Body Scan and related art project, 20 minutes plus cleanup

HOMEWORK:
Expand the Sai and the Horse story to events in your own life that might seem "good" or "bad" on first glance
Bring mindfulness to one physical movement you make regularly—brushing teeth, turning on faucet, walking, tying shoes, etc

Outline 3: More Sense Awareness

OBJECTIVES & KEY POINTS:
Bring greater awareness to senses
Awareness of relationships between perceptions, thoughts, and feelings
The power of looking deeply to become aware of what we usually don't see
Notice associations we have—the creation and formation of thoughts and feelings from perception

MATERIALS:
A number of objects with distinct smells—foods, spices, plants, earth, pencils
Paper and pencils

ACTIVITIES:

Sound Awareness, 15–20 minutes (p. 62)
What the Nose Knows, 15–20 minutes (p. 39)

HOMEWORK:

Three mindful breaths whenever you hear a phone ring, door close, car horn, or some other sound. Best if children all agree on one and engage their families.

Day 4: The Body in Motion, the Body at Rest

OBJECTIVES & KEY POINTS:

Teach children greater awareness of their bodies in motion
Importance of body awareness
Ways to deal with boredom by looking inward rather than outward
Mental and physical benefits of relaxation
Have children take pulse before and after practices
Learn to tolerate boredom and impulses
Learn to teach the body to relax

MATERIALS:

Enough space to lie down, walk, move, stretch

ACTIVITIES:

Boredom and Impulse Meditation, 10 minutes (p. 110)
Walking Meditation, 10–15 minutes (p. 87)
Ice, Water, Vapor, 15 minutes (p. 60)

HOMEWORK:

Take mindful breaths when at the bottom of a stairwell, and practice walking up first few steps mindfully
Take one breath before speaking when you can remember

Day 5: Loving Kindness Practices

OBJECTIVE & KEY POINTS:

Learn to have compassion for each other

Become aware of the body's signals about physical boundaries with others

Learn about the importance of relationships

Kids who don't feel comfortable hugging can just do the gazing portion of this exercise

MATERIALS:

Either colored construction paper, prayer flags, or squares of stiff cloth, string, permanent markers

ACTIVITIES:

Hugging Meditation, 10 minutes (p. 40)

Prayer Flags: Each person in the group gets a prayer flag, offers positive feedback or wishes for someone else, and writes them on the flag. Kids can take their flag home, or you can hang them where you work.

Outline for a Teen Group

Day One: Introductions

OBJECTIVES:

Understand stress

Clarify definitions of meditation and mindfulness

Learn purpose of meditation and mindfulness

Practice mindful awareness through exercises

Learn basic posture

Learn to use the breath as an anchor for practice

Key Points:

First, it is important to review the basic expectations. Then continue with some explanations of stress, and the idea that stress is about not being in the here and now, but rather about being in the future (next week's test), the past (reliving last week's embarrassment), or in another place (wondering what that boy or girl thinks of me). Then go on to explain that meditation practice and mindfulness practice in particular allow us to get in touch with the present moment, and with that simple act, stress begins to dissolve. Use the snow globe metaphor to demonstrate a clear, settled mind in contrast to a stormy mind, reminding students that perfect clarity is impossible, but more clarity is definitely possible.

Older kids will have a sense of what meditation is, either from their parents or popular culture. Ask them what they know, encourage them to share, and gently correct any misconceptions. It can be helpful to explain that meditation is not turning off thoughts; you may want to invite kids to try this for several minutes and show how impossible it really is, and then remind them that mindfulness practice is about watching thoughts and watching our experience so that we can come to know it.

Activities:

Eating Meditation, 20 minutes (p. 76)

Sitting and Lying Down Meditation, 5 minutes plus discussion (p. 11)

Homework:

Five minutes of sitting each day using breath awareness

DAY 2: Body Awareness

Objectives:

Learn the significance of mindful body awareness

Practice body awareness exercises

Insight into relationship between sensation and thought
Learn to use the body as an anchor for practice

Key Points:

Wisdom of the body, that when we pay close attention to sensations, we can come to watch how our thoughts and emotions also arise, linger, and eventually drift away

Benefits of knowing your body for health, athletics, and other things it does for us

Parallels between emotional and physical discomfort and the ways we can learn to tolerate them, the urges that arise with them, and the simple truth of their impermanence

Activities:

Body Scan (p. 93)
Walking Meditation (p. 87)
Points of Contact (p. 58)

Homework:

Make one body movement mindful. That can be the first two blocks of your walk to school, putting on your clothing in the morning, or the fine movements involved in brushing your teeth (doing this with the nondominant hand can really help bring attention to the task)

Continue to sit, using breath or body as anchor

DAY 3: Sound and Thought Awareness, Relaxation

Objectives:

Learn to notice sounds that exist in the silence, events that arise when we deeply listen or pay attention deeply

Learn to fully relax the mind and body and allow it to care for us

Become familiar with breath awareness

Learn to use the breath as an anchor for practice

KEY POINTS:

Mindful sound awareness has clear parallels to mental awareness and mindfulness meditation of just watching thoughts as they arise

Learn to relax and engage the mind and body in this

Understand that relaxing is different than distracting

ACTIVITIES:

Sound Awareness, 25 minutes (p. 62)

Riding the Waves, 15 minutes (p. 71)

HOMEWORK:

Practice riding the waves or listening to sounds for a few minutes first thing in the morning, and right before sleep. Some kids like to make signs and put them on their bed to remind themselves.

Continue to sit, using breath or body or sounds as anchor

DAY 4: Sitting and Loving Kindness

OBJECTIVES:

Sitting for longer

Learning loving kindness

KEY POINTS:

The group now has practice and experience with three anchors: the body, through body scans and anchor awareness; the breath, through practice of Riding the Waves; and sound awareness, through the Six Senses exercise. When sitting, they can now practice whichever feels most comfortable.

ACTIVITIES:

Metta Meditation (p. 15)

Begin with a longer sitting period (10–15 minutes or longer depending on your group), in which the group can use sounds, body awareness, or the breath as an anchor. Begin a guided metta meditation (p. 15).

HOMEWORK:

Write your own metta verses and send them to strangers on the street or around school

DAY 5: Retreat Day

OBJECTIVE:

Longer periods of practice, bringing mindfulness to our daily living

ACTIVITIES

Walking meditation for 5 minutes
Sitting for 5 minutes
Eating for 15 minutes
Finish metta for 10 minutes
Discussion and closing ritual

There are many possibilities for closing rituals. Some ideas include having the group share their favorite qualities of each person in the group by writing these down, or perhaps making wishes for each other on prayer flags. What is important is to honor each individual and give them something to take home and treasure.

Using Technology to Sustain a Practice

One of the many wonderful aspects of meditation is its simplicity. We need nothing but our breath and body, and for thousands of years practitioners used little else. Today it can be easy to fall into the trap of spiritual materialism, seeking out the perfect cushion, bell, and yoga pants. It truly can help our practice to have a comfortable cushion the way a good pair of running shoes can help an athlete, but we must be mindful that such things do not distract us from our intentions.

Technology is not going anywhere, and we as adults can wring our hands in concern about the damage we worry it is doing to young minds, or we can learn to adapt it and make it a positive force in our children's lives. I have found technology to be helpful in engaging kids and in building community—making technology useful rather than the distraction we can worry it will become. For starters, there are countless computer and smart-phone applications that will serve as meditation timers and even ones that can be set at random intervals throughout the day. These can be found easily with a quick Internet search.

What I think is the most exciting use of technology is in the communications that have resulted in creating freedom and pathways to freedom throughout the world. A world of people practicing mindfulness is out there, and they are online, sustaining and enriching each other's practice. You can join them and allow your more mature students to join up with others. Running a mindfulness group at Tufts University last fall, we were able to use the Internet to our advantage in just this way. We used the educational website Blackboard to post readings about the course, sound files of guided meditations, and tips for practice. But the communication was bidirectional, of course, and students also used the discussion space to post their experiences and share other websites and resources they had found. The group went on to form a Facebook Sangha and remain in touch, gently reminding each other to return to their breath.

Our goal for the future is to record the groups so that others can follow along at their own pace if they can't make our once-a-week time. Blackboard is an educational package, but many blogging sites offer free space for posting information, discussions, and even sound files. Recording yourself guiding meditations, whether you post them online or just make copies for people, will help your students make the bridge from the group to practice on their own, ultimately internalizing the meditations for themselves. We posted audio downloads on the counseling center website and handed out CDs at outreach events. We even set up a dial-a-meditation dedicated phone line with short meditation instructions in English, Spanish, and Korean. Soon we are adding Portuguese, Dutch, Hindi, and more languages as students volunteer to record them.

Another exciting computer-related development is in the area of biofeedback and neurofeedback. Programs and equipment that teach breathing and relaxation techniques can be bought for less than a few hundred dollars. Sensors placed on the hands communicate with the computer to visually represent progress toward relaxation and other mind and body states. Get creative and stay open-minded! Who knows what technologies we'll have by the time you are reading this book!

Appendix 2
Mindfulness Resources

Online Meditation Resources:
Iamhome.org
Innerkids.com
Dharma.org
Dharmapunx.org
Self-compassion.org
Mindandlife.org
Meditationandpsychotherapy.org
Mindfuled.org (Mindfulness in Education Network)

Retreat Centers in the United States:
Spirit Rock – Woodacre, CA
Insight Meditation Society – Barre, MA
Barre Center for Buddhist Studies – Barre, MA
Insight LA – Santa Monica, CA
Cambridge Insight Meditation Center – Cambridge, MA
New York Insight Meditation Center – New York, NY
Blue Cliff Monastery – Pine Bush, NY
Deer Park Monastery – Escondido, CA
Shambhala Mountain Center – Red Feather Lakes, CO

Family Resources:

Faber, Adele and Elaine Mazlish, *How to Talk So Kids Will Listen & Listen So Kids Will Talk* (New York, NY: Harper Paperbacks, 1999).

Greenland, Susan Kaiser, *The Mindful Child* (New York, NY: Free Press, 2010).

Kabat-Zinn, Myla and Jon Kabat-Zinn, *Everyday Blessings; The Inner Work of Mindful Parenting* (New York, NY: Hyperion, 1997).

Klass, Perri and Eileen Costello, *Quirky Kids: Understanding and Helping Your Child Who Doesn't Fit In* (New York, NY: Ballantine Books, 2004).

Levine, Noah, *Dharma Punx* (San Francisco, CA: HarperOne, 2004).

MacLean, Kerry Lee, *The Family Meditation Book* (Boulder, CO: On The Spot Books, 2004).

Murdock, Maureen, *Spinning Inward: Using Guided Imagery with Children for Learning Creativity & Relaxation*, (Boston, MA: Shambhala Publications, 1987).

Books for Children and Teenagers:

Hesse, Hermann, *Siddhartha* (New York, NY: Bantam Classics, 1981).

Loundon, Sumi, *Blue Jean Buddha: Voices of Young Buddhists* (Boston, MA: Wisdom Publications, 2001).

Muth, Jon, *Zen Shorts* (New York, NY: Scholastic Books, 2008).

Nhat Hanh, Thich, *The Dragon Prince* (Berkeley, CA: Parallax Press, 2007).

Nhat Hanh, Thich, *A Pebble for Your Pocket* (Berkeley, CA: Parallax Press, 2010).

Tezuka, Osamu, *Buddha* (New York, NY: Vertical, Inc., 2006).

Winston, Diana, *Wide Awake: A Buddhist Guide for Teens* (New York, NY: Perigee Trade, 2003).

Mindfulness Books For Adults:

Barks, Coleman, *The Essential Rumi* (San Francisco, CA: HarperOne, 1995).

Chödrön, Pema, *When Things Fall Apart: Heart Advice for Difficult Times* (Boston, MA: Shambhala Publications, 2002).

Germer, Christopher and Sharon Salzberg, *The Mindful Path to Self-Compassion: Freeing Yourself from Destructive Thoughts and Emotions* (New York, NY: Guilford Press, 2009).

Goleman, Daniel, *The Meditative Mind* (New York, NY: Penguin Putnam, 1988).

Henepola Gunaratana, Bhante, *Mindfulness in Plain English* (Boston, MA: Wisdom Publications, 2002).

Kabat-Zinn, Jon, *Full Catastrophe Living: Using the Wisdom of Your Body and Mind to Face Stress, Pain, and Illness* (New York, NY: Delta Publishing, 1990).

Kornfield, Jack, *A Path with Heart: A Guide through the Perils and Promises of Spiritual Life* (New York, NY: Bantam, 1993).

Kornfield, Jack, *The Wise Heart: A Guide to the Universal Teachings of Buddhist Psychology* (New York, NY: Bantam, 2009).

Levine, Noah, *Against the Stream: A Buddhist Manual for Spiritual Revolutionaries* (San Francisco, CA: HarperOne, 2007).

Nhat Hanh, Thich, *Happiness* (Berkeley, CA: Parallax Press, 2009)

Nhat Hanh, Thich, *The Miracle of Mindfulness* (Boston, MA: Beacon Press, 1999).

Sakyong Mipham, *Turning the Mind into an Ally* (New York, NY: Riverhead Books, 2004).

Siegel, Daniel, *The Mindful Brain: Reflection and Attunement in the Cultivation of Well-being* (New York, NY: W. W. Norton Company, 2007).

Suzuki, Shunryu, *Zen Mind, Beginner's Mind* (New York, NY: Weatherhill, Inc., 1970).

Williams, Mark et al., *The Mindful Way through Depression* (New York, NY: Guilford Press, 2007).

Spiritual Stories:

Fronsdal, Gil, *The Dhammapada: A New Translation* (Boston, MA: Shambhala Publications, 2005).

Kornfield, Jack and Christina Feldman, *Stories of the Spirit, Stories of the Heart* (New York, NY: HarperCollins, 1991).

Psychotherapy and Professional Books:

Baer, Ruth A., ed., *Mindfulness-based Treatment Approaches* (Amsterdam, NL: Academic Press, 2005).

Benson, Herbert, *The Relaxation Response* (New York, NY: Quill,1975).

Epstein, Mark, *Thoughts Without a Thinker: Psychotherapy from a Buddhist Perspective* (New York, NY: Basic Books, 1995).

Germer, Christopher K., et al., *Mindfulness and Psychotherapy* (New York, NY: Guilford Press, 2005).

Hayes, Steven, *Get Out of Your Mind and Into Your Life: The New Acceptance and Commitment Therapy* (Oakland, CA: New Harbinger Publications, 2005).

Linehan, Marsha, *Skills Training Manual for Borderline Personality Disorder* (New York, NY: Guilford Press, 1993).
Schoeberlein, Deborah, *Mindful Teaching and Teaching Mindfulness: A Guide for Anyone Who Teaches Anything* (Boston, MA: Wisdom Publications, 2009).

Acknowledgments

A WISE FRIEND once told me that when you achieve one of your goals, it's easy to be proud but important to be grateful. Whatever we do, we never do it alone. With that, there are so many people and teachers I would like to thank. So many beings working together across time and space contributed to the creation of this project that I have been able to assemble. But there are also specific people in my life to whom I wish to express my gratitude for their contributions to this project. First and foremost: my original committee, who helped bring this vision to fruition. Thank you for your patience and dedication, especially in the face of fires, blizzards, and sudden medical complications, even death. Thank you for your early commitment to the research that eventually became *Child's Mind*: Stephanie Morgan, Jean Bellows, Ethan Pollack, and Janet Surrey.

Thanks to my parents for introducing me to meditation at a time in my life when I needed saving from darkness. You planted the seeds and taught me to water them. You have supported me in this and my other projects and endeavors throughout my life, encouraging and gently suggesting. Olivia, thank you for your support, patience, open-mindedness, and ruthless editing. Thank you to my sister Mara for your support.

There are numerous meditation and Dharma teachers I would like to acknowledge my debt to (and theft from). In rough order of exposure: Jon Kabat-Zinn, Doug Phillips, Thich Nhat Hanh, Bill W., Dr. Bob (and all your friends), Pema Chodron, Jack Kornfield, His Holiness the Dalai Lama, Bill Alexander, Elaine Loechner, Estelle Simons, Henepola Gunaratana, Noah Levine, Robert Hall, Paul Fulton, Sumi Loundon, Narayan Liebensen-Grady, and Susan Kaiser Greenland. Thank you to

Chris Germer for your guidance in the publishing world, and thanks to the entire Institute for Meditation and Psychotherapy for building a path so many years ago. Other teachers and mentors have inspired me as well: Rhonda Sabo, Ron Wagner, Mike Elkin, David Trimble, Ted Sutton, and of course Kris, Peter, Darby, CL, Jason, and Mike.

My wonderful academic mentors also include Jill Bloom, Hal Cohen, and so many others. My supervisors over the years have also always encouraged and nurtured my passion for this topic: Julie, Linda, Ed, Ayanna, Diana, Rhonda, Vicki, Mohuidden Ahmed, and Leigh.

My friends and colleagues have also been extremely supportive, with particular thanks to Jen Dotson, Bill O'Brien, Cathy Glenn, and Eben Lasker for their support and encouragement. Co-workers like Stacey, Allison, Allyson, Erik, Lynn, and others have offered great feedback as well. And thank you so much to all volunteers and staff from the IMS teen retreat. Thanks of course to Ben, Stephen, the Superfriends, and Chuck, plus of course my group of friends here in Boston—Anne, Ariel, Gabe, Ben, and Carlene. There are more than I can name.

Of course, thank you to Rachel Neumann, and all of Parallax Press for believing in this project and nurturing it to fruition. Finally, I would like to recognize the suggestions and hard work of my students and patients these past few years, teaching me more than you are probably aware of and showing me that this stuff really does work.

Notes

1 Dieter Vaitl et al., "Psychobiology of Altered States of Consciousness," *Psychological Bulletin* 131 (1999): 98–127; B. Rail Cahn and John Polich, "Meditation States and Traits: EEG, ERP and Neuroimaging Studies," *Psychological Bulletin* 132 (2006).
2 Daniel Goleman, Destructive Emotions: A Scientific Dialogue with the Dalai Lama (New York, NY: Bantam, 2003).
3 Deborah Rozman, Ph.D., Meditating with Children (Buckingham, VA: Integral Yoga Publications, 1974).
4 Christopher K. Germer, *Mindfulness and Psychotherapy* (New York, NY: Guilford Press, 2005).
5 Jane Wexler, The Relationship Between Therapist Mindfulness and Therapeutic Alliance (Boston, MA: Massachusetts School of Professional Psychology, 2006.)
6 Cahn and Polich, *Psychological Bulletin* 132.
7 Germer, *Mindfulness and Psychotherapy*.
8 Cahn and Polich, Psychological Bulletin 132.
9 Herbert Benson et al., "The Relaxation Response," *Psychiatry* 37 (1974).
10 Cahn and Polich, *Psychological Bulletin* 132.
11 Jon Kabat-Zinn et al., "Part II: Influence of a Mindfulness Meditation-based Stress Reduction Intervention," Constructivism in the Human Sciences 8 (2003).
12 Richard J. Davidson et al., "Alterations in Brain and Immune Function," *Psychosomatic Medicine* 65 (2003).
13 Adapted from Lorin Roche, Meditation Made Easy (San Francisco, CA: HarperOne, 1998).
14 Adapted from William and Susan Morgan, "Cultivating Attention and Empathy," *Mindfulness and Psychotherapy* (New York: Guilford Press, 2005).
15 Steven C. Hayes, "Acceptance and Commitment Therapy and the New Behavior Therapies," *Mindfulness and Acceptance* 33 (2004).
16 His Holiness the Dalai Lama, from the Wisdom Commons Website (www.wisdomcommons.org), 2010.
17 Inspired by a Jack Kornfield story.
18 Adapted from Lorin Roche, *Meditation Made Easy*.
19 Adapted from Kimberly Rowe, *A Settled Mind* (Cumberland County, ME: Five Seeds, 2005).
20 Adapted from Lisa Desmond, *Baby Buddhas* (Kansas City: Andrews McMeel Press, 2000).
21 Inspired by Ajahn Chah and Maureen Murdock.

22 MarkWilliams, John Teasdale, Zindel Segal, and Jon Kabat Zinn, *The Mindful Way through Depression*. (New York, NY: Guilford Press, 2007).

23 Deborah Rozman, Ph.D., *Meditating with Children* (Buckingham, VA: Integral Yoga Publications, 1974).

24 Adapted from Robert Hall.

25 L. J. Harrison, R. Manoch, and Katya Rubia, "Sahaja Yoga Meditation as a Family Treatment programme for Children with Attention Deficit-Hyperactivity Disorder." *Clinical Child Psychology and Psychiatry* 9 (2004).; R. Semple et al. and Ruth Baer in *Mindfulness-based Treatment Approaches* (Amsterdam: Elsevier Academic Press, 2006).

26 Julie Brefczynski-Lewis, et al., "Neural Correlates of Attentional Expertise in Long-term Meditation Practitioners," *PNAS* 104 (2007); Lazar et al., "Functional Brain Mapping of the Relaxation Response and Meditation," *NeuroReport* 11 (2000); G. Pagnoni and M. Cekic, "Age Effects on Gray Matter Volume," *Neurobiology of the Aging* 28 (2007); and Cahn and Polich, *Psychological Bulletin* 132.

27 D. Chan and M. Woollacott, "Effects of Level of Meditation Experience on Attentional Focus," *Journal of Alternative and Complementary Medicine* 13 (2007); D. Foris, "The Effect of Meditation," *Journal of Undergraduate Research* VII (2005).

28 S. C. Hayes, "Acceptance and Commitment Therapy and the New Behavior Therapies," V. M. Follete et al., *Mindfulness and Acceptance, Expanding the Cognitive-Behavioral Tradition* (New York, NY: Guilford Press, 2004); Rozman, *Meditating with Children*; Daniel Goleman, *The Meditative Mind* (New York, NY: Penguin Putnam, 1988).

29 Adapted from Marsha Linehan.

30 Jon Kabat-Zinn, "Mindfulness-based Interventions in Context," *Clinical Psychology: Science and Practice* 10 (2003).

31 Jon Kabat-Zinn et al., "Compliance with an Outpatient Stress Redction Program," *Journal of Behavioral Medicine* 11 (1988); J. Kabat-Zinn, *Clinical Psychology: Science and Practice* 10; Daniel Goleman, *The Meditative Mind*.

32 Benson, *The Relaxation Response* (New York, NY: Quill, 1975); C. R. Schneider et al., "Behavioral Treatment of Hypertensive Heart Disease in African-Americans," *Behavioral Medicine* 27 (2001); R. Vyas et al., "Effect of Meditation on Respiratory System, Cardiovascular System and Lipid Profi e," *Indian Journal of Physiology and Pharmacology* 46 (2002).

33 To make origami boats that work even better, go to www.origami-fun.com/origami-boat.html or www.origami-instructions.com/origami-boat.html.

34 Laurie Keefer, "The Effects of Relaxation Response Meditation on the Symptoms of Irritable Bowel Syndrome," *Behavioral Research and Therapy* 39 (2001), Laurie Keefer, "A One Year Follow-up of Relaxation Response Meditation on the Symptoms of Irritable Bowel Syndrome," *Behavioral Research and Therapy* 40 (2002); D. Morse, "The Effects of Stress and Relaxation on Oral Digestion," International Journal of Psychosomatics 32 (1985).

35 J.L. Kristeller, Ruth Baer and R.W. Quillian. "Mindfulness-Based Approaches to Eating Disorders.," in Ruth Baer, ed. *Mindfulness and Acceptance-based Interventions* (San Diego, CA: Elsevier Press, 2006).

36 L. Roemer et al., "Incorporating Mindfulness and Acceptance-based Strategies in Treatment of Generalized Anxiety Disorder," *Mindfulness-based Treatment Approaches*.

37 Susan Morgan, "Turning toward Life," in Germer, et al., *Mindfulness and Psychotherapy*.

38 K. Lambert, "Rising Rates of Depression in Today's Society," *Neuroscience and Biobehavioral Reviews* 30 (2006).
39 C. Hammen and K. Rudolph, "Childhood Depression," in E. J. Mash & R. A. Barkley, *Child Psychopathology* (New York: Guilford Press, 2005)
40 Susan Morgan, "Turning toward Life."
41 Zindel Segal et al., *Mindfulness-based Cognitive Therapy for Depression* (New York, NY: Guilford Press, 2002).
42 Marsha Linehan. *Skills Training Manual for Borderline Personality Disorder*, (New York: Guilford Press, 1993).
43 J. M. G. Williams et al., "Mindfulness-based Cognitive Therapy Reduces Overgeneral Autobiographical Memory in Formerly Depressed Patients," *Journal of Abnormal Psychology* 109 (2000).
44 Adapted from Steven Hayes.
45 James Blumenthal et al., "Exercise and Pharmacotherapy in the Treatment of Major Depressive Disorder," *Psychosomatic Medicine* 69 (2007).
46 Anna M. Tacon et al., "Mindfulness Meditation, Anxiety Reduction, and Heart Disease," *Family and Community Health* 26 (2003).
47 Adapted from Thich Nhat Hanh.
48 Asian folk Tale adapted from Jack Kornfield, *Roots of Buddhist Psychology* (1996).
49 Anna Marie Albano et al., "Childhood Anxiety Disorders," in E. Mash and R. Barkley (Eds.), *Child Psychopathology* (New York, NY: Guilford Press, 2003).
50 Germer, *Mindfulness and Psychotherapy*.
51 Baer. *Mindfulness-based Treatment Approaches*.
52 Adapted from Maureen Murdock.
53 Adapted from Jon Kabat-Zinn.
54 Sonya Batten, Susan Orsillo, and Robyn Walser., "Acceptance and Mindfulness-based Approaches to the Treatment of Post-traumatic Stress Disorder," in Orisllo and Lizbeth Roemer (eds.), *Mindfulness-based Treatment Approaches* (New York, NY: Springer, 2005).
55 V. M. Follette et al., "Acceptance, Mindfulness and Trauma," *Mindfulness and Acceptance* (New York, NY: Guilford Press, 2004).
56 Batten et al., *Mindfulness-based Treatment Approaches*.
57 Lizbeth Roemer et al., "Incorporating Mindfulness and Acceptance-based Strategies in Treatment of Generalized Anxiety Disorder," in *Mindfulness-based Treatment Approaches*.
58 E. R. Valentine and P. L. G. Sweet, "Meditation and Attention," Mental Health, Religion and Culture 2 (1999); Benson, *The Relaxation Response*.
59 Jon Kabat-Zinn et al., "Part II: Influence of a Mindfulness Meditation-based Stress Reduction Intervention," *Constructivism in the Human Sciences* 8 (2003).
60 Julie Brefczynski-Lewis et al., *PNAS* 104.
61 Noah Levine, *Against the Stream* (San Francisco, CA: HarperOne, 2007).

Parallax Press, a nonprofit organization, publishes books on engaged Buddhism and the practice of mindfulness by Thich Nhat Hanh and other authors. All of Thich Nhat Hanh's work is available at our online store and in our free catalog. For a copy of the catalog, please contact:

Parallax Press
P.O. Box 7355
Berkeley, CA 94707
Tel: (510) 525-0101
www.parallax.org

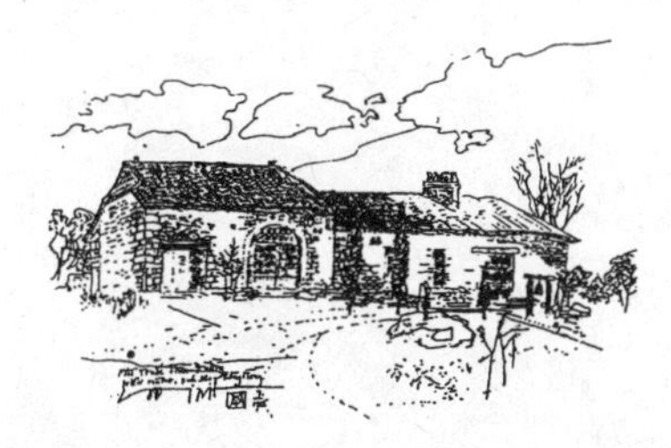

Monastics and laypeople practice the art of mindful living in the tradition of Thich Nhat Hanh at retreat communities worldwide. To reach any of these communities, or for information about individuals and families joining for a practice period, please contact:

Plum Village
13 Martineau
33580 Dieulivol, France
plumvillage.org

Magnolia Grove Monastery
123 Towles Rd.
Batesville, MS 38606
magnoliagrovemonastery.org

Blue Cliff Monastery
3 Mindfulness Road
Pine Bush, NY 12566
bluecliffmonastery.org

Deer Park Monastery
2499 Melru Lane
Escondido, CA 92026
deerparkmonastery.org

The Mindfulness Bell, a journal of the art of mindful living in the tradition of Thich Nhat Hanh, is published three times a year by Plum Village. To subscribe or to see the worldwide directory of Sanghas, visit **mindfulnessbell.org**.